Reconceiving Black Adolescent Childbearing

Reconceiving Black Adolescent Childbearing

Elizabeth Merrick, Ph.D.

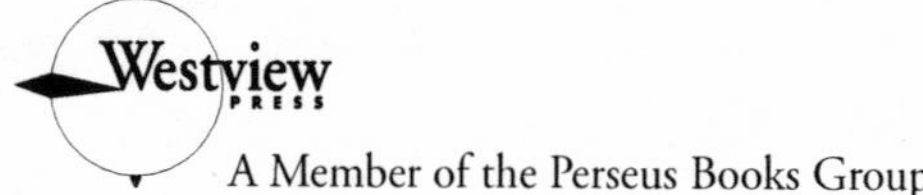

A Member of the Perseus Books Group

Published in 2001 in the United States of America by Westview Press, 5500 Central Avenue, Boulder, Colorado 80301-2877, and in the United Kingdom by Westview Press, 12 Hid's Copse Road, Cumnor Hill, Oxford OX2 9JJ

Find us on the World Wide Web at www.westviewpress.com

Library of Congress Cataloging-in-Publication Data
A CIP catalog record for this book is available from the Library of Congress.
ISBN: 0-8133-6816-2

The paper used in this publication meets the requirements of the American National Standard for Permanence of Paper for Printed Library Materials Z39.48-1984.

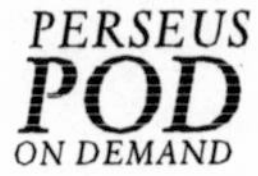

10 9 8 7 6 5 4 3 2 1

Contents

Acknowledgments

The young women who participated in the study deserve primary acknowledgment. Without their willingness to share their experiences, this research would not have been possible. This project was assisted by many people at different stages. In writing the book, I received invaluable feedback and support from Barbara Launer, Sallie Motch, Mary Sue Richardson, and Lisa Simon. I was also aided by the comments of an anonymous reviewer at Westview. Finally, I was fortunate to have the unflagging support of my husband, Sam, who with our children, Lizzie, Charlotte, and Sam, provided the incentive and encouragement necessary for me to finish.

1

Introduction

I used condoms with every partner that I had except my baby's father. I don't know why I didn't use it with him. Well, to tell you the honest truth, I wanted to have his child, I did. That's the only reason I didn't use it. . . . And I always wanted to have a child. But it just happened.

—*Edouine*

Images of pregnant black teenagers and single black mothers are plentiful in the media and popular culture. These representations have fueled debates on the need for welfare reform and have focused public attention on adolescent pregnancy among black Americans. However, the pervasive focus on black adolescents tends to obscure the facts that the rates of black adolescent childbearing are at their lowest levels to date and that white adolescents are having babies in much greater numbers.[1] Media portrayals of the phenomenon tap into middle-class beliefs about indiscriminate, promiscuous sexual activity as well as judgments of these young people's disregard for their futures and those of their babies. On the one hand, these representations feed into middle-class fears about welfare abuse: that many are "getting more than they should." On the other hand, these images simultaneously serve to confirm beliefs that these unwed adolescents, and their offspring, "get what they deserve" as they remain trapped within limited circumstances. The relationship between adolescent childbearing and poverty—as both an antecedent and a consequence—is often an explicit concern.

The unwed black welfare mother—typically envisioned as a teenager or as a woman who began her childbearing as a teen—has emerged as a powerful stereotype. The "face" of adolescent pregnancy is assumed to be black in discussions of what ought to be done about the problem and in the minds of most Americans. (This assumption, Luker points out, is both true and not true. It is true in the sense that rates among black adolescents are disproportionately high,[2] however it is not true, statistically speaking, given that the majority of births to adolescents are to white teens.) Beliefs about adolescent childbearing, including those related to "race," have been challenged by social construction theorists.[3] Their critiques highlight the influence of social context and suggest that our current understandings of the "problem" of adolescent pregnancy are rooted less in "fact" and more in public sentiment. Such perspectives do not suggest that there is no problem, or that the problem has been socially constructed in all aspects. However, these critiques raise important questions about how the issue of adolescent pregnancy has been framed.[4] In addition, Phoenix (1993) and others[5] have directed attention to how the issue has been constructed along racial lines.

It is important to note that the issue of black adolescent childbearing has been largely constructed by mainstream white society. The national dialogue about adolescent childbearing featuring poor black adolescents is conducted about—and not with—those involved. Thus, although adolescent black women are typically the subject of discussion and the target for intervention efforts, the perspectives of pregnant black adolescents of lower income are absent. This omission contributes to their continued marginalization[6] in spite of their visibility as stereotypes. In this void, pregnant black adolescents are typically depicted as irresponsible pursuers of sexual pleasure or as manipulators seeking to profit economically through having a baby. To a lesser degree, these young women are sometimes portrayed as "children having children" or as victims themselves.[7] Although several researchers have conducted ethnographic studies with adolescent black mothers (e.g., Kaplan, 1997; Williams, 1991), there is a need to engage with pregnant black adolescents' perspectives on their pregnancies and childbearing to seek their own descriptions of their views and their situation.

This book addresses this void by presenting the stories and voices of six pregnant black adolescent girls whose stories I sought in a qualitative study on childbearing.[8] The bulk of the book consists of the stories of these young women, with whom I conducted ethnographic interviews attempting to understand their pregnancies through their eyes. Although these young women were not selected as a "representative" group, their stories present a variety of perspectives that stand in contrast to popular stereotypes about pregnant black teens. Indeed, what becomes foreground, when listening to these young women, is how very human, and adolescent, their struggles are. Engaging with their perspectives, and their lives, provided direction toward a reconceptualization of black adolescent childbearing. This reconceptualization is rooted in their beliefs or philosophies about their lives.

I began the study with an interest in learning about the participants' views of their pregnancies and childbearing. My original questions reflected my focus on learning the circumstances surrounding becoming pregnant. However, as part of the method, I also anticipated that my questions would change in response to what I learned. Early in the course of interviewing, the realization that their views of their pregnancies and childbearing were inextricably linked to their life experiences and beliefs about life led me to widen my focus to include learning their personal histories and views.

The findings that emerged were complex and led me to grapple with questions about agency or the extent to which they had "chosen" pregnancy and childbearing. In making sense of the findings, I struggled to appreciate the strong contextual factors that influenced their childbearing while acknowledging their individual agency. In doing so, I relied on works from feminist psychology[9] addressing issues of power and control as well as works from black women's psychology[10] dealing with resistance and accommodation.

The widening of the research lens beyond a focus on "adolescent childbearing" also led to a consideration of the participants in terms of their development. In contrast with views that address adolescent pregnancy as a "problem behavior," childbearing is seen here to be one, inextricably linked part of a larger picture of the young women and their lives. Knowledge of the development of ethnic minority and economically disadvantaged teens is limited. However, an emerging body of research suggests that the realities of life for adolescents within lower-socioeconomic-status (SES) urban black communities contribute to developmental trajectories that differ from those of majority youth (Burton, Allison, & Obeidallah, 1995).[11] Here, I argue that adolescent childbearing represents an alternative developmental pathway for some young women.

Issues of development and agency are threads that run throughout the book. As a context for the consideration that follows, I provide an introduction to these issues. I first review and critique understandings of adolescent development. I then address the connection between adolescent childbearing and poverty and summarize three current explanations of black adolescent childbearing. In considering these explanations, an essential question is addressed: whether, or how, a focus on black adolescent childbearing is warranted. In the remainder of this chapter, I describe the research study.

Adolescent Development

At first glance, this study's focus on childbearing among black adolescent girls seems consistent with a long tradition of literature that addresses lower-income, urban minority adolescents in terms of "problem behaviors" such as pregnancy, substance use, and failure to complete school.[12] In general, limited attention has been devoted to studying adolescent development among minority youth; in particular, there are large gaps in our knowledge about urban minority adolescent girls' development (Leadbeater & Way, 1996). As a result, there has been a sustained call for work that explores a range of minority youths' lives and behaviors and attends to differing contextual demands and outcomes (Bell-Scott & Taylor, 1989; Jessor, 1993; Zaslow & Takanishi, 1993).

Common understandings of adolescence as a time of transition between childhood and adulthood reflect an awareness of the biological and social factors that mark the second decade of life (Feldman & Elliott, 1990). Although certain physical changes associated with puberty may signal an individual's entry into adolescence, the social markers that help to define adolescence are less clear and are dependent on societal expectations.

Theories of development traditionally identified specific tasks to be achieved during adolescence. Successful resolution of these tasks presumably led to a more autonomous, individuated, and independent self. Erikson's (1968) theory, for example, emphasized an adolescent's struggle for autonomy that Erikson defined as "the courage to be an independent individual who can choose and guide his own future" (p. 114). Although decades of research and intervention efforts were guided by theories such as Erikson's, traditional assumptions about the tasks and processes of adolescent developmental theories have recently been challenged. Particular criticism centers on the fact that most traditional theories of adolescent development are based on understandings of white, typically male, middle-class youth (Gilligan, 1982; Taylor, 1994). As a result of this bias, development among women and others whose developmental experience varies from this norm has frequently been defined as lesser or deviant (Taylor, 1994).

Recent research with varied populations has led to a reconsideration of assumptions about seemingly universal conceptions of adolescence and human nature (McHale, 1995). In particular, adolescence does not seem to be the clear developmental stage it was assumed to be (Burton, Obeidallah, & Allison, 1996; Jessor, 1993). Researchers note that the separation of the achievement of adult status from sexual maturity and the emergence of an extended period of dependency (often institutionalized through schooling for mainstream youth) are relatively recent, Western developments (Arnett, 2000; Hill, 1999). Other theorists, including Irvine (1994) and Modell and Goodman (1990), note the historically and socially constructed nature of the meaning of adolescence.

Critics of traditional understandings of adolescent development have also cited the limits of a Eurocentric framing of tasks and processes of child and adolescent development. Hill (1999), for example, has argued the need to include tasks such as racial socialization and gender role socialization, among others. In addition, a major area of contention relates to the assessment of developmental outcomes. Researchers have argued that traditional measures typically fail to capture developmental achievement among diverse youth. Attempts to remedy this situation are preliminary and controversial.[13] However, recent research supports the importance of evaluating adaptation in context given the demands and constraints of a lower-income environment (Winfield, 1995).

Adolescent Childbearing and Poverty

Recent scholarly perspectives, including those of Luker, (1996); Dodson, (1998), and Musick (1993), suggest that poverty is a primary factor influencing adolescent childbearing. Persuasive evidence suggests that poor women, regardless of their race or cultural background, tend to have children young. Numerous studies correlate adolescent childbearing with variables related to poverty.[14] These variables include being raised in poverty, by a single parent, with a low level of education. Life experiences associated with poverty are thought to influence early childbearing by lowering the perceived cost: Impoverished youth may see there is little to lose by early childbearing given their limited experience of alternatives. In addition, recent research[15] suggests that the consequences of adolescent childbearing may not be as negative as previously thought, particularly among lower-income individuals. Several longitudinal studies of lower-income black women suggest that initial differences may be made up over time (Furstenberg, Brooks-Gunn & Morgan, 1987) and that early childbearing may offer relative advantages such as the provision of a family network for child care (Geronimus & Korenman, 1990).

Current scholarly perspectives, such as those of Luker (1996), Dodson (1998), and Musick (1993), that forward poverty as the primary factor influencing adolescent childbearing do not address black adolescent childbearing as a special case. The traditionally higher rates of black adolescent childbearing are assumed to be attributable to the higher rates of poverty among black Americans. The movement toward subsuming black adolescent childbearing under a larger umbrella of adolescent childbearing appears to be a mixed blessing. On the one hand, an understanding of adolescent childbearing based on poverty tends to shift the terms away from "race" toward more "universal" class terms. Given the negative ways in which black adolescent childbearing has been traditionally, and tragically, miscast as a issue of "culture,"[16] this seems like an appealing move. On the other hand, a highlighting of the influence of poverty to the exclusion of other factors dismisses a voluminous body of scholarly work on the unique sociocultural factors particular to black Americans that may influence early childbearing.[17] A review of three current explanations of black adolescent childbearing reveals important differences in the framing of the issues involved.

Cultural Perspectives

In sorting out whether or how black adolescent childbearing warrants a separate focus, it seems essential to begin by engaging with the perspectives of black women and black feminist scholars.[18] Although no consensus exists among black American women (or any other group), the works of selected black women scholars, including Collins (1990), Dickerson (1995) and Jordan (1992), among others,[19] offer important insights. These authors have critiqued white mainstream conceptions of black American single mothers. Their works contradict white views that have forwarded a simplistic understanding of the influence of poverty, or other "deficits" or "pathology," in framing an understanding of black lives.[20] Their perspectives identify the limits of applying traditional paradigms to understanding the phenomenon of black single motherhood and to understanding black women's experiences.[21] In doing so, they offer important directions toward a nonracist conceptualization of black adolescent childbearing.

A common thread among these works is the importance of acknowledging cultural factors unique to African Americans that influence their family forms. Many authors, including Dickerson (1995) and Sparks (1996),[22] have argued that the influence of West African heritage, including the importance of motherhood and community, is especially relevant. They posit that current family forms reflect the continuation of West African features, including the value of motherhood in the black community, an elaborate lineage system, and the significance of extended family. In addition, some theorists argue the creative and survival aspects of black American family patterns and forms. Jordan (1992), for example, acknowledges the strengths of black Americans against tremendous odds that include poverty.

In sum, these perspectives argue that the inclusion of cultural factors—either as a continuation of African heritage or as adaptations to racism and oppression—are essential to understanding black Americans' lives and family patterns. Critics of this point of view note that, in light of recent economic changes, the extended-family model may no longer be available to many black Americans.[23] In addition, this explanation fails to account for the strong disapproval of single parenting and adolescent childbearing within the black community (Hill, 1999; Kaplan, 1997; Ladner & Gourdine, 1984). Clearly, the situation is complex, and even proponents of this perspective have acknowledged limitations.[24]

Economic Perspectives

In contrast with cultural explanations of black adolescent childbearing, the economic explanation forwarded by Wilson (1987) argues that unwed black adolescent childbearing is due to economic and structural influences. Wilson's analysis focuses on economic shifts in the 1970s and 1980s that resulted in male joblessness in urban black communities. In Wilson's view, this factor, along with others, led to a dramatic decrease in the pool of marriageable (economically stable) black men that caused the rise of female-headed families and unwed adolescent childbearing. Although Wilson addresses "black adolescent childbearing" as an issue of the black community, he frames his arguments in terms of "class" not race.[25]

Consistent with Wilson's economic model, Anderson's (1990, 1993) ethnographic work focuses on the impact of economic and structural changes in an inner-city community. Anderson (1990), argues that black adolescent childbearing is "nothing less than the cultural manifestation of persistent urban poverty" (p. 113). Anderson's treatment of the relationship between "predatory young men" who lack an outlet for their strivings and young women who seek to "fulfill their dreams through pregnancy" rests on an economic assessment of the situation.

Criticism of Wilson's (1980, 1987) economic perspective comes from many directions.[26] In particular, critics have charged that his model reduces black adolescent childbearing to economic determinism and that his patriarchal view of the situation denies the influence of economic and structural factors on women (Kaplan, 1997; Polikow, 1993).

Gender, Race, and Class Perspectives

A third explanation of black adolescent childbearing is forwarded by theorists such as Brewer (1995), Jacobs (1994) and Kaplan (1997), who place gender, race, and class at the center of their analyses. Jacobs's (1994) study of adolescent mothers asserted the importance of girls' socialization, particularly within their families, in terms of gender, race, and class. In a similar vein, Kaplan's (1997) ethnographic study of two generations of black adolescent mothers identified the multiple intersecting influences of gender, race, and class on these women's lives and childbearing. Specifically, Kaplan (1997) argues that black adolescent childbearing is the result of a "poverty of relationships" that these girls suffer at adolescence.

Although these works are preliminary, they suggest exciting new directions for further research. One important issue that remains to be deeply addressed is that of agency.[27] Treatment of this issue seems essential to attempts to understand adolescent girls' experiences related to pregnancy and childbearing. A related weakness in this emerging body of work is that the research has been conducted exclusively with teen mothers whose views of their pregnancies and childbearing may be influenced by their after-the-fact feelings. Clearly, more theoretical and empirical work is needed in order to develop this perspective. In particular, this work should address the "interplay" between culture, economy, race, and gender (Brewer, 1995) and should shift the dialogue from a mainstream framing of the issues.

The Study

This book represents my attempt to understand pregnancy and childbearing from these adolescent black women's perspectives. I undertook the study with an aim, consistent with Collins (1990, 1993), to center my understanding of black motherhood on their perspectives. This attempt, however, is necessarily influenced by my identity as a white American woman of a middle-SES background. The implications of my "social location" in my perspective and this work are worthy of consideration. Some might argue that, given my identity, I cannot truly engage with their experiences,[28] and during the study, I grappled with this issue. However, I came to believe we can do good work about lives of others whose experiences we do not share and whose social location differs. Relying on Harding (1991), I believe I can only acknowledge and take responsibility for my social location. At all stages of the study, I worked to attend to the potential influence of my social location.[29] I have attempted to provide enough information for readers to determine whether my findings, and my interpretations of them, are legitimate.

This work grew out of my experience working as a counselor in an urban adolescent health center where the majority of clients were lower-income black American teens. As a counselor, I was struck by the discrepancy between the young women I encountered and the portrayals of adolescents like them in media images and in popular debates. In contrast with popular images, what I learned through my work with these adolescents indicated that the "reasons" for their pregnancies were not about welfare. Neither, for the most part, were they about ignorance or deviance. The picture was not what I would have expected given popular attention to the issue. The majority of those choosing to have children seemed quite reasonable in their assessments and their choice. Despite some naïveté in assessing the demands of parenting, most appeared to be making a choice that they felt would be best for them at this time in their lives and that seemed to have some normative value within their sociocultural context. I decided to pursue their stories in a rigorous way.

On a personal level, my desire to explore the discrepancy between "outsider" assessments and these young women's lived experience was fueled by my own experience. Growing up, assumptions about my family based on their educated, white, middle-class, and religious appearance had left little room for my own contradictory experience of my family. I knew firsthand the injustice done when superficial understandings exclude a more complex and challenging reality.

My own experiences of childhood trauma and abuse allowed me to connect with many young women's stories of hardship in ways that I could not have anticipated. As I listened to the young women I interviewed, I remembered my own tumultuous adolescence, and I often felt, "That could have been me." I connected with their struggles to create something better out of devastating circumstances, and I understood the possibility for hope in spite of these circumstances. My own decision, during the course of the study, to become pregnant provided opportunities for further reflection.[30] My sense of identification with some of the participants is in no way intended to lessen an awareness of the unique and important circumstances that mark their lives. Rather, an appreciation of the places where we are similar and different afforded a greater ability to learn and understand.

Method

I interviewed young women participating in the prenatal program of an adolescent health center where I worked as a counselor in a different program. This agency provides comprehensive services to a multicultural population aged twelve to twenty-one from the surrounding metropolitan area. Pregnant adolescents receive free health care and attend prenatal education classes. In order to obtain volunteers, I solicited participants from these classes a few times over the course of several months. Each time, I said that I was seeking to interview African-American[31] adolescents, who were around sixteen years of age, who were in their second trimester of pregnancy, and who had not previously given birth.[32] I told them that I was seeking to interview them because I wanted to know about their experiences and opinions about their pregnancies. I communicated to them that I was genuinely interested in what they had to say about their pregnancies and that I anticipated that their points of view might differ from those of an outsider.

I conducted in-depth interviews with six participants[33] who were included in this study. The use of a small sample is consistent with research that aims for depth in order to provide directions for tentative hypotheses and further research.[34] The primary purpose of ethnographic interviewing is to learn to see the world through the eyes of the person being interviewed (Ely, 1984). The interviews themselves contained questions intended to be open-ended, sensitive, and probing. Questions that guided the interviews at the beginning were usually broad "grand tour" questions (Spradley, 1979) through which I sought general information. In later interviews, I asked questions that were more focused and related to material presented by the participant. These questions were often about material we had discussed previously or about questions I had after thinking about the data.

I interviewed most participants four times each for about an hour each time over the course of weeks or months. I continued to interview them as many times as was necessary for elaboration or clarification of material from previous interviews and to check their views of the accuracy of my understanding of the data.

The analysis entailed an intense familiarity with the data. I initially achieved this by listening to the audiotape immediately following the interview and then listening again to the tape while reading the interview transcript. I then read and reread the transcripts, my notes, log entries, and analytic memos throughout the process of data collection and analysis. I sorted data in provisional categories and considered propositional statements to describe the data in each. For example, I initially tentatively proposed that "mothers seem important." I similarly developed themes that, as Ely et al. (1991) summarized, are statements of meaning that occur (1) frequently or (2) infrequently but carry heavy emotional or factual impact. These preliminary themes described the data within each category. These were written as first-person "I" statements," such as "I'm different from my mother."

When I interviewed each participant, I was concerned with learning about her particular story and pregnancy. At the same time, I considered each participant in light of what I had learned so far, and in terms of the overall findings for the group. After completing interviewing, I wrote first-person narratives to convey each participant's story and the major findings. The analysis and writing of the narratives furthered my analysis and understanding of data for the group; my analysis of the group similarly influenced the evolution of the individual narratives.

The study's findings are presented here in two ways: first, through the six narratives (presented in Chapter 2), which provide a profile of each participant and convey the major themes for each; then, through the themes (presented in Chapters 3 through 6) that emerged as shared or significant from my analysis of the data. The presentation of the themes contains examples from the data using material from the participants' interviews. Following each theme, or group of themes, my discussion is presented in the form of a "Reflection." In each reflection, I address related literature. In Chapter 7, I focus on several seeming contradictions in the thematic findings discussed in Chapters 3 through 6. In Chapter 8, I address implications for an alternative developmental model based on these pregnant black adolescent girls' perspectives.

Notes

1. The National Center for Health Statistics (NCHS, 1999) reported that the birthrate among unmarried black teens has fallen 20 percent since 1991. *National Vital Statistic Reports* (1999) indicated that there were 340,894 births to white teens aged fifteen to nineteen and 219,292 births to black teens aged fifteen to nineteen.

2. Luker (1996) cites, "African Americans, who make up only about 15 percent of population of teenage girls, account for more than a third of all teenage mothers. And whereas six out of every ten white teenagers who give birth are unmarried, among black teenagers the ratio is nine out of ten" (p. 7).

3. These include Luker (1996), Nathanson (1991), and Phoenix (1992).

4. Luker (1996), for example, argues that this framing distracts attention from the underlying social and economic forces compelling young women to early childbearing.

5. These include Elise (1995), Sparks (1998), and Ziegler (1995).

6. Weingarten, Surrey, Coll, and Watkins (1998) define marginalization as a diminishing, or lessening, of experience in comparison with a prototype group—in this case, the prototype mother is married, heterosexual, neither "too young" nor "too old," etc.

7. In this perspective, pregnant teens are typically seen as passive or naïve victims who are often the prey of older males. The correlation of adolescent pregnancy with a history of sexual abuse is also noted.

8. A detailed description appears in Merrick (1995).

9. Davis and Fisher (1993); Fine (1989); and Mahoney and Yngvesson (1992).

10. Fordham (1993), Mirza (1992), and Robinson and Ward (1991).

11. See also Crockett and Crouter (1995).

12. See Jones (1989) and Leadbeater and Way (1996).

13. See Jessor, Colby, and Shweder (1996) for a summary of diverse positions on this issue.

14. See Coley and Chase-Lansdale (1998) for a review of psychological literature.

15. See Coley and Chase-Lansdale (1998).

16. In particular, the 'culture of poverty' perspective that identified black American family patterns as responsible for perpetuating poverty through transmission of values. See Sullivan (1988) for a treatment of this history.

17. These include Ladner's (1972) classic ethnographic study of girls approaching womanhood in a lower income black community and Burton's (1990) cross-generational ethnographic work suggesting that early childbearing may be part of an alternative life course strategy among lower-income black Americans.

18. Black men have also written about the issue of black adolescent pregnancy. However, their views are not engaged here.

19. These also include hooks (1981), Walker (1982), and Welsing (1991).

20. See Jordan (1992).

21. Scott (1991) and hooks (1981).

22. Elise (1995) also argues that the current characteristics of black American families reflect West African features.

23. See Anderson (1993), Jewell (1992), Kaplan (1997), and Wilson (1987).

24. See Dickerson (1995).

25. See Wilson (1980, 1987).

26. See Kaplan (1997).

27. While Kaplan (1997) acknowledges agency and its relation to structure, she does not address this issue in depth.

28. See Harding's (1991) discussion of pros and cons in her defense of the possibility of male feminists. One could also argue that, given the difference in social location, I might have been sensitive to aspects of their experience that would be missed by someone of the same location.

29. See Merrick (1999) for a description of the analysis process.

30. See Merrick (1995).

31. When I began the study, I chose to use the term *African-American* rather than *black* or *black American* because the latter seemed to refer to racial or physical characteristics rather than the ethnic or sociocultural similarities I sought. As the study progressed, it seemed the term *African-American* was not an accurate descriptive label since several participants described themselves as having mixed ethnic backgrounds. I subsequently dropped my use of the term *African-American* and determined that the race/ethnicity criterion would depend on how they self-identified, which, for most participants, was black or black American.

32. The reasons for these criteria are discussed in Merrick (1995).

33. I conducted initial interviews with five other volunteers; four of these did not meet the criteria for inclusion and one decided not to participate.

34. Guba and Lincoln (1989) and Lincoln and Guba (1985).

2

The Participants

This chapter contains findings in the form of six narratives. The narratives convey the major themes of each participant that emerged from the analysis of her interview material. The first-person narratives use the participants' interviews to convey what is most meaningful to them and to provide different participants' perspectives. In writing each narrative, I was guided by the question "What would a reader need to know about this young woman, her life, and her situation, to know her as I have through the research process?" Thus, the writing process also involved shaping the transcript material in order to communicate the participant's story clearly. In this, I made a significant effort to keep close to the character of the participants' dialogues. This shaping process is described more fully in Merrick (1995).

Each narrative begins with a brief description of the participant and her partner, and a summary of my interactions with the participants during the interview process. An introduction to each narrative contains a physical description of each participant that includes skin color because several participants discussed this as an important issue.

Kim

Introduction

Kim is a slender, seventeen-year-old light-skinned young woman who came to my attention when I presented my request for African-American participants to her prenatal class. She asked, "Can you only half-interview because I'm only half-black?" This initial remark revealed an intelligence, a sense of humor, and a tendency to test others' reactions that were evidenced in our subsequent interviews.

At the start of each interview, Kim often told me I would have to ask her specific questions. When I dodged this by asking what question she thought would be a good place to start, she came up with her own direction.

During the time we met, Kim was living with her mother, who Kim said was not supportive of the pregnancy. Kim was attending classes toward her high school equivalency diploma; she had been expelled from a private school when they learned she was pregnant. Kim said she was hoping to begin college sometime after she had the baby.

Kim described having conflicted feelings about her partner, Colin. She said that he was twenty-three and was involved in the music industry and in some things that could be dangerous, which she couldn't discuss. Kim said that she was trying to adjust to the fact that he had other girlfriends and children and that he was only minimally involved with her and the pregnancy.

Narrative

When people who know me from before find out that I'm pregnant, they can't believe it. People weren't expecting this. I guess because I've been in private schools all my life—from little Catholic schools to the bigger ones like Burgess. I was raised in that whole academic thing and I had a very strict and controlling mother. My mother did everything for me, and my life is supposed to go according to her direction. She raised me to believe that you go to school, you go to college, you get a job, you get married, and then you have children. And nothing can get in the way of that—you have to stay on that path.

My mother basically did everything for me because my mother's Asian, she's Chinese. Chinese are very manipulative people, they really are. I mean, they will choose out your path, and they'll tell you what to do. You don't have a real relationship with your parents. They think that they're doing enough by giving you a home and paying for it. But that's not enough—I've always wanted more. I wanted love.

My mother was there, but she wasn't there emotionally if you know what I'm saying. When I needed her, when I had a lot of problems, she just didn't understand. Instead of helping me, she'd say, "When I was seven, I was out in the rice fields with my sisters." Because that was her life growing up in China. She couldn't relate to me and my life here. The differences between us are because of age and also because of culture. My mom thinks that Western society is very twisted compared to China. She thinks because I'm Western, I'm spoiled and petty. She's also never liked that I'm different from her in terms of looks and other things.

When I was growing up, my father did catering and bar-tending and my mother was a housekeeper. She still does that—cleans house for rich white folks. When I was born and when I was younger, we were living in a mostly poor black neighborhood. We had a slum lord and we didn't have hot water—that was disgusting. We weren't exactly poor, on welfare, or anything. But my father had a lot of bills 'cause he was very sick and he was old, so we weren't financially wealthy.

My father died when I was twelve and he was seventy-four. He had diabetes and two kinds of cancer. My whole life, my younger life, I was in hospitals all the time. I think that really messed me up mentally. It was very stressful. Nothing about my life was very normal because of having a sick, older father and because I'm part Chinese and black. People would look at me differently and stuff because I didn't exactly look like one or the other.

I think it also messed me up that my mother didn't know how to raise a black American child. Like when it came to my hair, she'd just say, "Ugh, your hair." She didn't really know what to do with it. Once in a while, the girls in my neighborhood would go and braid my hair for me. But other times, my mom would just end up cutting off all my hair so I had an Afro. She did that twice; that's why I don't let her touch me, ever again, when it comes to hair and other things.

Growing up, I had to rebel a lot because I never really got to do anything I wanted to do. I started having a life, a social life, and having a sexual life that she didn't know about. That started when I was about fifteen. And I didn't think school was that interesting. It was so easy for me that I started hanging out more and more. That's how I met Colin, the baby's father.

When I met Colin, I was going out with this other guy who was really nice, but who I didn't get to see that much. So I started hanging out downtown. Colin definitely made an impression on me right away. I don't believe in love at first sight, but it was just something about him. I got into a conversation with him and we just started talking. From then on, I basically ended up going to see him whenever I could. We became close on a mental level and we would talk about a lot of things.

He said he was nineteen when I met him, but he just turned twenty-three. I guess he said he was nineteen because he could get away with it. He also told me he was staying at his sister's, but I figured out later that he actually stays with his girlfriend, Tamika.

Colin's a wonderful storyteller. After we started having sex, a few times I asked him where the condom was. He didn't have any and I would ask him if he wanted me pregnant. He would say, "Yeah, yeah." So, I said, "Fine." I think he would say anything to shut me up.

Getting pregnant is partially my fault. I will admit that; I didn't really do much to prevent it. I wasn't always protected. I mean if I was really against getting pregnant, I would've used something. I mean it's not like I set out to try to get pregnant, but whenever I'd have sex, I'd think, "What's going to happen with us? What if I got pregnant?" And with Colin, I thought it was different.

I guess it was different because I started to think that I could have his baby. With guys before, I thought I couldn't have a baby from them because they were knuckleheads. But somehow it was different with Colin. I mean, he's always been a knucklehead and he always will be a knucklehead. But I had very strong feelings for him.

At the time I got pregnant, I was kind of going downhill, not really caring about myself. I wasn't really sure about the future or whether I even cared about the future. I was hanging out, drinking and smoking. I was with this girl who hung around drug dealers and I was even smoking weed. So, I was hanging out more and doing stupid and crazy stuff, out of frustration and depression. A lot of things just bring me down. When I get like that, I usually don't have the strength to actually pull myself up.

Usually I rely on other people. That's why I'm using this baby—to pull myself up. Meaning that I actually have something to live for. I have something to look forward to, something to work for. Because when it comes to myself, I don't really have enough ambition.

When I found out I was pregnant, it wasn't a good time for me. I was pretty down; I couldn't get out of it. I was emotionally empty. Colin and I were fighting, and he was taking advantage of me and having other girlfriends. When I told him I was pregnant, he tried to make me have an abortion. He said it was because he knew how hard it would be for me to deal with my mother. But I thought it was because he just didn't want to have a baby with me.

When I told my mother, she freaked out and said she was going to kick me out of the house. She told me I should have an abortion. Early on in the pregnancy, I thought about it and I wasn't sure what I was going to do. One day, I was coming home from school, feeling down. And I was thinking, "I guess I'll have an abortion 'cause it'll be so hard to have a baby." But when I came home, my mother was talking on the phone, telling her friend all about the pregnancy. They both tried to tell me to have an abortion. It made me so mad! Here she was talking about my business to someone unimportant and trying to tell me what to do! I'd had it. So I just said, "I was going to get an abortion, but now, forget it, I'm not."

Adults tend to disregard that kids actually have brains and use them. If we think that something's not right, we do just the opposite. Just to show you it's not right, if you know what I'm saying. You say, "Mommy, I'm seventeen years old, why do I have to be home at eleven?" And you'll come home at twelve o'clock just to piss her off, just to show her that you're able to take care of yourself.

People often say teenagers having babies are doing it to be independent. In a way, it's true. I don't think it's right to have a baby just to prove you're gonna do something your mother doesn't want you to do. But it's like that for me. I'm having this baby to be independent. My mother thinks I'm gonna have the child and dump it on her. She says that I better not expect her to take care of it. I don't. This pregnancy isn't my mother's decision, this is *my* responsibility. I mean, I'm not asking her to like it, I'm just asking her to be there for me. This pregnancy is my responsibility and something *I* want to take care of.

That's another reason why, when I thought about having an abortion, I couldn't do it. I think it would be like having a big piece of me removed, cut out. They might as well cut out my heart. I would feel like a big piece of me would be missing, like I'd be alone again. To me, it would be stopping a new life—my life, my new life, of doing things and taking responsibility. Things are different now.

Now that I'm pregnant, I actually know what I want to do, I actually know what career I want. It's much more clear now. Before, college always seemed scary because I never had that much ambition. I was scared to leave for college; I wasn't sure I could take care of myself. That's what I was afraid of. But now, it's different. Before, I could have said that I wouldn't need to eat for a week, but I can't say that now. I can't say that my baby will go without diapers for a while. There are things I have to do for the baby.

Before, when I was in school, I didn't really know what I wanted to do. That was because I just thought what I'd been trained to think, what my mother told me. She raised me that you finish high school, you go to college, and then you get a job. The reason it wasn't clear was because it wasn't my path. Those were my mother's plans for me, not mine. So how could I fill in the details? Now that I'm pregnant, I know that I'm hopefully going to stay in the city and maybe go to a city college. I want to take a liberal arts curriculum in sociology and then get my M.S.W. and something will hopefully come from that.

On the one hand, I'm thinking about the time when I'll come out smelling like a rose, when I finish college and get my master's in social work. But, on the other hand, I worry. I don't know how I'm going to do all that without money. I know I'll have to get a job and I've never had a real job. Once in a while, I've packed bags at the supermarket, but that wasn't a real job. I don't know what I'm going to do. I don't even know if I'm going to get welfare. It's very confusing. I know I need money. I hope Colin will be able to get me money, at least for the basic stuff like a crib. And I want my kid to look good, too.

I have faith that in the back of his mind Colin knows what's right. I hope that he'll come around and be there for me. But I'm not going to rely on him, though, because he would get upset at that. I could make all these plans, but they don't include him because I can't count on him. I can't say that he will marry me and pay for my college education and everything. I'd like to, but I know I can't do that. You can't plan what another person is going to do. But if it happens, if he does help out, then it will make my life easier.

Even though I know I can't count on him, I still can't help but daydream. I daydream that one day Colin will fall in love with me again and take care of me and the baby and forget about all the other girls. These are just daydreams though, and sometimes I have to tell myself that this is not going to happen. My mind still keeps doing it, though. I guess it's to make me feel better. I'm not really sure. Maybe it's to make me feel less abandoned. I feel less alone if I think that maybe one day he will get his act together. It's just daydreaming, though; we'll see what happens.

Right now, I'm living day-to-day but I'm also living toward a future goal. I want to have a healthy child and to have enough money to do things. And I want to do better on my SAT this time. Those are my goals. Right now, my mother's disappointed in me, she thinks that my life is over. Basically, I believe my life will be over once I give up on myself—and I'm not giving up!

Edouine

Introduction

Edouine is a slight figure. She has coffee-colored skin and her features seem overpowered by a pair of thick-lensed glasses. She has an open smile and a quick, friendly manner that makes her seem older than sixteen. She speaks easily in a quiet but intense voice with a slightly southern accent.

Edouine's partner, Khary, is twenty-four. She said she tries to see Khary whenever she can; he is in jail and in a work release program. Edouine was upset about this and hoped he would be out by the time the baby came.

During her pregnancy, she was attending a program to get her high school equivalency diploma. Edouine was living with a friend and sometimes stayed with her grandmother.

Edouine was easily involved in the interview process. We met five times, and our interviews often ran more than an hour. Edouine said that it was different for her to talk about herself, and that she enjoyed it. She said she sometimes stopped by to see if I was in just to talk.

Narrative

I didn't know how to tell my mother I'm pregnant because my mother's alcoholic. If I tell my mother something like that, she just goes to the liquor store and gets drunk. I didn't want to tell her 'til she was out of the shelter. My brother told her, and she's happy about it. She says she can't wait 'til the baby's born. She was fifteen when she had her first child, so I knew she wouldn't be complaining about me being pregnant.

My mother's been drinking all her life and my grandparents didn't trust her around me. They took me away from her when I was a year old, after my father died. I don't know much about my father but I always say he must've been a sweet man to put up with my mother. After he died—he was shot—I've been with my grandparents. Well, I lived with them until I was fifteen, when my grandfather died. Then I moved from place to place. I stayed at my brother's, and then I moved back with my mother. We stayed in a shelter until she got too outrageous with the alcohol. I left her and went to live with my friend. Now I live with my friend and sometimes I stay with my grandmother.

I think I would go insane if I lived at my grandmother's all the time. My grandmother is too religious—she's a churchgoing person and she's strict. We'd go to church on Tuesdays, Fridays, and Sundays, and sometimes Saturdays. My curfew is at 10:30 or 11:00 and my grandmother wants to know where I'm at every minute. She's too strict, so I just don't stay with her too long.

My grandmother was the one who raised me, though. Her opinion goes a long way with me because I respect her. She clothed me, she fed me, she put a roof over my head, and I can't disrespect that. But I know she's upset with me. Every time she looks at me, she's got to eat. That hurts me; I know why she's eating. She ain't hungry; she's just disgusted with me. She'll look at me and start crying. She's upset that I'm pregnant, and it makes me feel bad.

I hope things change, because I can't have my grandmother being bigger than me! Even though she's upset, my grandmother told me, "No matter, you're having a baby, I'm here for you if you need me. If you ever need some money or whatever, I'm here." I'm glad because I can't really depend on my mother. It's just me by myself and then my grandmother.

When people found out I was pregnant, a lot of them said something about my age—I'm going to be seventeen. My grandmother felt a tad embarrassed because she's a church person. People are looking down on her because they say it was her responsibility to keep me out of the sex zone, that's how they put it. But at the time I got pregnant, I wasn't living with my grandmother, they should know that. If I was, I know I wouldn't be pregnant now. I wouldn't because she's so strict.

When I got pregnant, I was living at my best friend's house. I had left my mother and she was living in the shelter because she was drinking. My boyfriend, Khary, used to come over a lot to visit. Me and him used to do what we have to do, nice and all. My friend's mother was not all that strict. She felt it was better for me and her daughter to do it in the house instead of doing it somewhere on the street because that ain't for young ladies. Or doing it in a back seat of a car, that ain't for young ladies either. She thinks it's better if she knows where we at, and she knows that we safe.

The father of the baby, Khary, he's twenty-four; he's real nice. He's a sweet guy and he takes care of his kids. The baby's father got three kids. He's there whenever the kids need something. A lot of people think he's irresponsible. Sure, he is irresponsible if he got three kids by three different women, and then he going to have a fourth child by a fourth woman, and he lives with one of his babies' mother.

A lot of people and my grandmother say it's wrong. They say that I don't know what he's doing, and when the baby is born he's not going to be there. They may be right; I don't know because right now, he's in jail. I don't know when he's going to come out. I hope he'll be out by the time the baby comes. I don't know what he did and I don't want to know because that would stress me out even more.

I don't know why my baby's father wanted me pregnant. It's not like it's his first child. Sometimes, I feel like I'm in fourth place. I think that once he takes care of the first one, takes care of the second one, takes care of the third, by the time he comes down to mine, he won't have no money. And his list probably goes on and on, with more after me, knowing him.

What attracted me to him? He made me laugh. Every time I was down and sad or had a problem I could always talk to him. He was like my brother more than my boyfriend. We was more buddies than boyfriend and girlfriend. He made me laugh. If you can't make me laugh, I'd be depressed all the time. We were together five months before I got pregnant.

I used condoms with every partner that I had except my baby's father. I don't know why I didn't use it with him. Well, to tell you the honest truth, I wanted to have his child, I did. That's the only reason I didn't use it. I thought that he would make a good father. I thought, "He's there for his other kids, let's see." And I always wanted to have a child. But it just happened.

I love kids. I always wanted to see a little me running around the house. So I could say, "Look at my daughter," and I would be proud. And I want one of my own to see how I'm going to raise it. To see if I'm gonna raise it different from the way my grandparents or my mother raised me. I don't want my kid to be raised up the way I was raised up or to drop out of school like I did. I want them to be different than I was, in a lot of ways, because my life was terrible.

When I was thirteen, I just realized I have to take care of myself because nobody else is going to do it for me. Ever since then, I do everything for myself. Whatever I want, I get it for myself. I try to do things by myself. And if I can't do it, I'm not going to worry about it.

I've felt that way ever since I found out what my mother was all about. Since I realized that she didn't . . . my mother loved me, but in a little way she don't love me because of being alcoholic. My mother could be a little tipsy and say some shocking things to me. I'd think, "You ain't drunk yet, how can you say this to me?" My mother says things that make you feel like she don't care.

I know a lot of people feel like I'm not like my mother and I'm glad. I don't want to be like her. I don't want to be an alcoholic, have my man beating up on me, and people taking advantage of me, people spending my money, and me getting kicked out from place to place because of something silly.

My mother dropped out of school in the fourth grade. She started drinking early and just dropped out. And she'd tell me, "Get up and go to school." And I'd say, "But did you go?" She'd tell me, "Don't play with me." And I'd say okay but I'd go right back to sleep. I would tell her, "You should make yourself an example. You know, finish school, get a job, whatever. Don't sit home being lazy." I used to always say that. She'd be telling me, "You need a job," and I'd say, "But do you got one?" I used to get her all the time. My grandmother would tell me to stop it. And I'd say, "But she didn't do it. And she's my mother. How can she tell me something if she didn't do it herself?" That's the way I'd always put it to my grandmother. My grandmother said, "But you don't do what she does. You want to be smarter and intelligent and have a good job and she's going to sit home looking like a bum and an alcoholic." So I'd feel like that was true and I'd get up and go to school.

I want to finish school so that when my child asks me if I went, I can say that I finished all twelve grades, well, to eleventh grade and got my GED. And tell my child I'm working at a job or college. So then my child would say, "If my mother can do it, I can do it."

When I think about the future, I know I want to finish school and have a good job. That's important to me. I know it will be hard. I want to finish school, go to a year of college, then get pregnant again. After the older baby is about three years old and in nursery school, then I'd go back to work. I'd want to have a morning or a day job. And at night, I'd have my child and a nice house or an apartment.

I want to go to law school. I'm striving for law school because I'd like defending people. I think about how a lot of people get off scot-free killing. I think if you killed a person, you should do the time in jail. And sometimes innocent people go to jail; there's proof that they didn't do it but they don't use it. I would love to do that; I'd like defending people. Plus, my family says I can lie real good so they tell me I'd make a good lawyer. I can lie real good 'cause I was the youngest and I always got blamed for everything. If something got broken or whatever, I'd keep track of it so I didn't get blamed.

I think if it's meant for me to be a lawyer, it's going to happen. Whatever happens, happens. If I wind up working somewhere, I just wind up working there. If I don't, I don't. If it happens, it was meant to be; if it wasn't, it wasn't. It's like when me and Khary was together, it wasn't like we were trying to have a baby but we said, "If it happens, it happens." The baby wasn't meant to be, but maybe it was. So, if it's meant for me to be a lawyer, it's going to happen.

In school, they told me that as long as you try your best and do what you can do, you can get what you want. They told me, "Don't let nobody tell you that you can't do it. Because if you let somebody tell you that, you'll never get nowhere. You've got to be your own person." That's the way I feel about it and that's what I'll try to do.

I just wonder what's going to happen down the line as I grow older and maturer. I wonder if I'm going to be the way I am now, always friendly and considerate to other people's needs and helping other people. Or will I just be looking out for myself?

My grandmother feels that people are going to run over me and that I won't have any money. But I told her when that time comes, I'd know how to walk away from it. She tells me, "You're too smart, you're too smart." My grandmother always told me that every time I speak, I speak with maturity. She says that you'd never think that I'm just going to be seventeen. A lot of people think I'm older. They ask, "How do you know so much?" I say, "Because I've been there. I'll be seventeen, but I've been there. People running over me, people throwing me out their house, men doing this and that to me, everything. I've been there."

Chantel

Introduction

Chantel is eighteen and wears her hair pulled back in a pony tail. She has dark skin and a solid figure. She dresses neatly in matching shorts and shirt sets. She wears no jewelry except a small diamond-type ring on her left hand—an engagement ring from her partner, Stephen.

Chantel had graduated from high school and was in her first semester of college when she got pregnant. Stephen, the father of the baby, occasionally comes with her to the clinic. He is nineteen, works at an office job, and is in the military reserves. Chantel lives with Stephen and his mother. She had been living in a group home for two years before that and has no contact with her family.

We met four times for about forty-five minutes each time. At the start of each interview, Chantel often yawned and looked pained. She seemed not to want to be interviewed but, when asked, said it was okay, that she was just tired. After I offered her tea and cookies and we ate, she seemed to relax and talked easily and at length.

Narrative

When I was coming up, I grew up with neither parent. I was put in foster care when I was three weeks old. My father would come visit at the foster care agency, but he didn't want me. Legally, I was given to him at five but he didn't want to keep me. So I stayed with a foster family, but they weren't my foster family legally. When my natural father finally did come into my life, when I was about nine, he was abusive. He used to come on the weekends and take me for weekend visits. He blamed me for problems between him and my mother, and he was disappointed that I wasn't a boy. When I was about nine, he started becoming physically abusive. My foster mother turned alcoholic at the same time. So, actually, I had nowhere to turn.

It seems like I've always been rejected. When I was coming up, I felt rejected. There I was, three weeks old, being put into foster care, rejection number one. Then when the courts gave me to my father when I was five years old, and he didn't want me, rejection number two. Then when I needed to be supported by somebody, when I needed somebody in my life, there was nobody there—my foster mother's alcoholic, my father's abusive, rejection number three.

I'm eighteen now, so most of my life I've been rejected. I've always wanted somebody to love me; I've always wanted to be loved. That's why I feel like now, when this baby comes, I can just love this baby and this baby can love me. I know this baby won't judge me; it's too young to judge me. The baby will accept me for who and what I am, not for the other things that people judged me for when I was younger. I don't really know what my father and my mother judged me for; I just know they didn't want me. But I know I can't be rejected by this child because this is my child.

I'm happy that I'm having the baby because I feel like I can get so much from this child as far as love is concerned. And I'd be able to love it back. It's not like I'm just in it for myself. I'm in it for the baby, too. I want to give my love to somebody now, other than my boyfriend, if you know what I mean—somebody that's actually related to me, like family, somebody that has my blood.

My whole life I never really had any family. I mean, I don't love my father; he doesn't love me. I don't love my mother, my natural mother; she doesn't love me. I have brothers and sisters and we all have the same mother but different fathers. And I just met them; I didn't grow up with them.

I have one other sister, Nola, who's younger, who I've never met. She was adopted right after she was born. I heard that she looked like me and I've always wondered what she's like. I have this fantasy that someday I'll write to Sally Jessy Raphael or Oprah and they'll reunite us. It would be like finding that missing link. I'm going to name my child, if it's a girl, Nola, after her.

My mother's had so many children, each with a different father. It seems like my mother was having children and nervous breakdowns left and right. My mother is crazy; I should say mentally ill. She's mentally ill legally. She's been hospitalized a lot. I didn't spend that much time with her when I was growing up, but whenever I did—it was scary. She asked me one time, "How about if your mother was Jesus?" I was so scared because I was alone with her. She was like on the edge of a nervous breakdown. I didn't stay with her too often.

When I was thirteen, my father finally wanted to take me. And I became a runaway because I couldn't stay with him. He was so mean, he'd lock me in the house and threaten me and other things. So, I ran away and was staying with friends and in shelters. I was moving back and forth, from place to place. That was until I went into the group home when I was sixteen, where I was stable for the last two years.

When I was in the group home, I started wanting to have a baby. I guess it was because I'd see other people with babies and they made it look so nice. I know it's hard, but they make it look so nice—so lovey-dovey, like they're really in love and they're really happy. I started thinking that I wanted a baby, I wanted somebody to love me.

In the group home, two girls got pregnant, and I thought, "I want to be like them." They moved out of the group home and went to a mother-child residence. I figured they were probably just having babies to get out of the group home. And I felt that wasn't right, that they shouldn't use a baby like that. I could understand it, though. I'd wanted out of the group home from when I was sixteen years old. You're allowed to stay until you're twenty-one, but I decided that at eighteen I would be out. It was hard living there with all the rules and regulations. There's a lot of stress living in a group home.

That's why when Stephen, my boyfriend, came along, I wanted to take advantage of the situation. I was thinking, "He really loves me; let me kinda like hop on this. This could be my ticket out of the group home." In a way, I was using him, but I thought it could be good. So, I moved in with him and his mother.

Stephen is nineteen and I've known him for about three years. He's in the army reserves. We used to go together back when I was fifteen, but we broke up and I didn't see him for about two years. He said he never forgot me, and last summer we started going out again as friends. All the time I was in the group home, I had been celibate. I hadn't had sex with anyone for two years. I knew that if I was going to have sex with somebody, I was going to do it because they loved me and I loved them. Once I got back with Stephen, I knew we loved each other. We got engaged in the winter, and a month later I got pregnant.

Stephen had talked about wanting to have a baby. I had told him, "What makes you think I'm going to have your baby?" I don't really know how it came up. I think he must have mentioned it when we were talking about getting married because we had just gotten engaged. He asked me, "How many kids are you going to have?"

We had used condoms all the times we had had sex before. But after we had been talking about having a baby and saying that we wanted one, we didn't use one when he was home on leave in December. And when I got my menstruation, I asked him if he was mad. The next month, I even counted the days. I know ovulation occurs fourteen days from the beginning of your menstruation. It starts after about fourteen days; that's when you're the most fertile. And then it's like two days prior to that and two days after that you can get pregnant. So I was making sure we did it on those days and everything. This time it was on purpose; we were trying to have a baby on purpose. But for some odd reason, I just didn't think that it was going to happen.

I just didn't think that I could be pregnant. It was like, "Nah," you know, "my period's probably just late." I don't know why. Conception just seems so complicated. Because it's like when a man ejaculates, sperm has to go through a little tiny, microscopic hole in the cervix. Then it swims, and some of them don't make it, la, la, la, and finally one gets to it, and you know. I was like, it couldn't happen. That couldn't happen to me.

When I found out I was pregnant, when I first told Stephen, we had had a fight and we weren't speaking. I have to say we fight a lot, and we get into physical fights. When I told him I was pregnant, it was like talking to a brick wall. He just looked at me, gave me this cross-eyed look, and kept writing or whatever. He just said, "Well, do whatever you want to do." Like I could have an abortion! At that moment, when I felt like I didn't have his support, I felt like "I don't believe this." I was flabbergasted. "Now what?" I felt so torn apart emotionally. I couldn't believe it.

I told him I was going to get an abortion. And I got back at him the only way I knew I could—I beat him up. When I beat him, he finally acknowledged how I felt. He said, "Let's just slow down and stop fighting." Then we talked about it and he let go of the anger. He told me that I couldn't have an abortion, that he wanted the baby. I felt like, "Thank God, I have his support."

Even though I told Stephen I was going to have an abortion, I don't think I could've done it. I thought about it, but I just couldn't do it. I feel like I'm already emotionally shot from all the things that have happened in my life. I mean I've been through a lot already. I've taken a lot of stress, and I'm still taking on a lot of stress. So I felt that having an abortion would just be loading on more stress. Having an abortion would make me even worse.

And when I thought about abortion, I started thinking about how my parents were. I thought, "If I have an abortion, I'd be rejecting this baby. That's just like my parents." That's what I felt like, even though a lot of people say it's just a fetus. I said, "How could I?" I would feel guilty for the rest of my life. I don't think I could've done it. I don't think I would have made it through mentally.

There were times in my life when I felt I was really going to go crazy. Sometimes I'd think I was on the edge of going really nuts, because of a lot of things that happened to me. Especially when I was fighting with my father. But then I'd think about the fact that I'm in college, that I have a lot of things behind me. I'd look at my grades—I have report cards with nineties and eighty-fives to show for what I did. So, that really backed me up. Education is the thing that always made me keep going. I mean, if you don't have an education, it's like you can't build yourself up. It's like, "What do I have? Nothing, I don't even have a high school diploma or a high-school equivalent."

I worked really hard in school. I went from high school to college without stopping. And every summer I went to summer school. So I never had any break. When I started college, I wasn't that excited; I was pretty tired of school. But I thought, "Let me just get started." I thought I wanted to be a police officer, that's what I was going to be. But then I changed my mind, and I wasn't sure what I should do. So, now that I'm pregnant, it's like I can think about what I want to do. Now, I have an excuse to be out of school to think about what I want. I still don't know yet, but hopefully soon I will find out. I think I want to go into like journalism or something like that.

After I have the baby, I'll probably go to school two days a week and still be a full-time student. Or I might have to go to night school with the baby if Stephen can't help out. If I have to carry my kid to school with me, then I'll do it. I will struggle for my child; I will struggle if I have to.

But my child will never know that we're struggling because he or she will be content. I will do everything to make my child happy.

Stephen and I disagree about that. Stephen said something that really pissed me off when I was three or four months pregnant. He said, "When you can't find a baby-sitter, send the baby to Trinidad." That's where he's from. That's what all them come up here and do. They have babies born here to make them a citizen of America and then they send them back to Trinidad with their relatives.

When Stephen said, "Send the baby away," I got so mad. I told him, "Why should I have somebody else raise my kid? This is something I got sick for." I told him, "You don't send a child away! You send mail away. You send a package away, you know, you send letters away. You don't send a child away!" I said, "Your momma sent you away to your aunt and your grandmother. And my parents sent me away to go live in foster care. Why in the hell, after I carried this baby for nine months, would I go send it away to somebody in Trinidad to raise my child?" I told him, "Hell no!" He better not ever mention that again.

That's something you just don't do! To me that's giving the child a message that you don't care. That's the message I got from my parents. And they sent me away when I was three weeks old! I feel that I would be doing the same thing to my child. My mother and father just sent me away. And I wouldn't wish that on any child.

Shamika

Introduction

Shamika is sixteen; she is small and looks somewhat athletic. She has dark brown skin, and she wears her short hair in barrettes and braids. She occasionally brought her nieces or her nephew with her to the health center and interacted with the children in a teasing, attentive manner.

Jamal, Shamika's partner, is seventeen and attends high school. Shamika said he writes and plays rap music with a group that has achieved some local success. When we began interviewing, Shamika was not attending school. She said she had been having trouble at her previous school and was planning to transfer. She subsequently enrolled in a school for pregnant girls. During her pregnancy, Shamika was living with her mother. She said that she and her mother were beginning to have a closer relationship.

During our interviews Shamika answered questions directly and briefly. She often yawned and seemed bored; however, when asked about this, she would laugh and respond playfully. After our third interview, Shamika learned that there was a genetic problem that would result in fetal demise and that she had to terminate the pregnancy. Shamika was clearly upset by this and had no contact with the clinic for several weeks. When she returned, she told me that, against medical advice, she and Jamal were trying to get pregnant again immediately. Her narrative is based on our first three interviews prior to the termination.

Narrative

I don't know how many weeks pregnant I am. I didn't figure I was pregnant because my period was coming. I wasn't thinking about it until my period only came for one day last month. But when I came to the doctor, he had me take a pregnancy test. I wasn't expecting to be pregnant, it just happened! At first when the doctor told me, I was a little surprised; then I just had to deal with it.

About three months ago, I had an abortion. So there was nothing on my mind like I could be pregnant again. When I told Jamal, my boyfriend, that I was pregnant again he was surprised, too. That's sort of shocking—that it could happen just three months later. I didn't know it could happen that soon. I thought it would take a little time for my body to get back together after the abortion.

The first time I got pregnant, I wasn't using birth control. I knew about it but I wasn't taking nothing, because I thought that it couldn't happen to me. That's what I wanted to believe. I thought maybe if I thought like that hard enough it wouldn't happen, but it did.

When I got pregnant that time, I had an abortion because it was unexpected. Things just weren't going right between me and Jamal. We were having a lot of problems. I had other boyfriends and I was with somebody else. That baby's father was acting up, saying he didn't want the baby, that it wasn't his. When I told Jamal about it, he said that I should do whatever I wanted to do and that he'd be there. But I didn't feel comfortable keeping it. I feel that if the father ain't gonna be there from the start, it don't need to happen. So I had the abortion.

My first experience of abortion, I didn't like it. Before I went and had it, I never saw anything about abortion. But as soon as I had one, it was hard to forget. It seemed like everything was just reminding me of it every time I turned around! I kept seeing it on TV all the time and I saw commercials for the clinics on the train. I just got mad. I didn't like it. It made me sad. I decided that if I ever got pregnant again, I would keep it.

This time, when I got pregnant, I was on birth control pills. But I knew they wasn't gonna work for me 'cause they didn't work for my older sister or my mother. The pills aren't 100 percent effective. I had missed a day and took two pills the next day. I think that's when I got pregnant. Well, that happened a few times. I'd keep forgetting to take them or I'd be so sleepy that I'd fall asleep until the next morning. The pills could be looking me right in my face, and I'd say, "I'll take them in a minute." But then I'd forget.

When I found out I was pregnant this time, I told Jamal. We sat down and talked. He's the type of person that if he did it, he'll take responsibility for it. He just told me if I wanted to keep it that he'd stay with me. The decision about the pregnancy is really up to me. But it's both of our responsibility, so I think he should have a say-so. But if I didn't like his say-so, then I wouldn't do it! If he told me to have an abortion, I wouldn't go through it. So, in a way, he's important, but in a way, he's not.

If he decided that he didn't want to be bothered, I'd be prepared for it. I wouldn't get all emotionally upset and cry and want to give my baby away. Because when you're having a baby you gotta learn that the father might not always be there. You have to think that way nowadays because men just decide to pick up and leave when they want to. When they feel you're a burden, they could just decide to get up and leave.

My mother preaches and preaches about that constantly. That's because my sister's father left my mother. My grandmother also says that you have to be prepared. They both say that men can't really do nothing for you unless they got a job. My mother and my grandmother have been telling me this my whole life. They say, "The man won't always be there. He might not be able to do for you more than you can do for yourself." That's a saying from my great-grandmother: "A man can't do more for you than what you can do for yourself." They preach that you can do much more than a man can do, rather than sitting around waiting for a man to do it for you. They just keep saying it; that's how I know it. So, I'd be prepared if Jamal decided he didn't want to be there.

But Jamal's been there all the other times so I think I can take a chance with him. He's seventeen and he's in school. He and his two friends are in a rap group; they write songs and are getting ready to make an album. Jamal knew about pregnancy. He had got another girl pregnant. His mother used to ask him, "Are you using birth control pills, contraceptives?" He would say, "I don't like using those things."

I know Jamal had thought about pregnancy. He told me before that one day he wanted to have a baby. But I didn't know that he meant by me and right now! I think it kind of just happened. Because he didn't necessarily know I was going to get pregnant at that particular time. I think he wanted me to get pregnant, I don't know. Anyway, it's too late now, I just have to deal with it!

Jamal wants me to go to school 'cause he don't want no stupid baby mother. He's already said that. He said he'd stay home and take care of the baby so I could finish school. Or if he decides to work, he said that his mother would baby-sit.

School is really important to Jamal and to my mother, too. When I told my mother I was pregnant, she first asked me whether I was keeping it or not. When I told her I was keeping the baby, she just asked if I was going to still go to school. I told her I was. My mother is really concerned about education. As long as you go to school, she feels you can do anything in the world. And I know you can't do much without education, so I just have to really get serious in school now.

I'm trying to find a school that I'll be more comfortable in. I've had to change schools a lot because I have a lot of fights. Fighting's kind of normal for me. All the girls want to fight me because of boys. The first thing boys see about me is my eyes; my eyes look Chinese. When the boys see my eyes, they say, "Oh, she got pretty eyes!" and they want to be my boyfriend. The girls don't like that and they get mad and want to fight me.

People are always jealous of me. In my old neighborhood, where I used to live, people mostly wear Guess or Polo. When I moved, I was wearing that and people in my new neighborhood would say, "Oh, she got money," and they just want to fight me.

You *have* to know to throw your hands up! Or else you won't get nowhere. 'Cause once one person sees you can't fight, then everybody's gonna want to fight you. If I couldn't fight and some girl came up to me and I ran away from her, then all the girls that didn't like me already are gonna say, "We could just beat her up all the time." But in my projects where I live, all my cousins beat up most everybody in the projects. So nobody wants to mess with me. But I don't need nobody to help me out! Everybody in my projects knows I can fight.

Anyway, I hope I find a better school. One where I won't fight. Before it used to be hard for me to go to school. But once you're pregnant you just gotta think about things. That's what you do. I can't mess up in school because what kind of life will I have for the baby if I don't have a high school diploma. You have to ask yourself those questions.

I would like to do nursing or computers. I think about college but to get in those schools you have to have good grades and patience. In order to get good grades you have to stay in school all day long and go to class. I just want to go home. It's a drag when you have to carry your coat around all day long because you can't use the lockers. The school doesn't use lockers because of the drugs that people put in the lockers. So you gotta carry around everything. Every class has a book. When you get in the tenth grade every book is big!

I'll keep going to school after the baby's born. I don't think it'll be that different. I can't know what it's going to be like, but I don't think it's gonna be that bad. Like not all outrageous like some of these people make it sound. Like saying the baby will cry all night and cry all day.

They go on exaggerating. The reason babies cry a lot is because people spoil them. Like every time somebody comes in, they gotta pick the baby up or something. I know what's going to happen if you do that all the time. My first nephew, everybody picked him up all the time. He could be sleeping and somebody would pick him up. But, now he cries all night because he's used to somebody picking him up all the time. He still does that to this day. It's just pure spoiledness. There's no need for that. As long as he's clean, his diaper's changed, he's got his bottle, you showed him affection, what have you, that's all. I know because I have four nieces and a nephew. I've been through it all with them.

So I don't listen to what other people say about being a mother. Everybody's different. I just don't ask them. I'd just rather see for myself. If I made the biggest mistake of my life I have to deal with it. I'd just say, "Oh, well." I just thought about that one time and then I didn't think about it anymore. My mother just says I will see for myself. I don't ask her and she don't tell. She feels it's up to me, what I want. I chose it so I will just have to deal with it. That's the most important thing about pregnancy for me: Deal with it. It's too late now. 'Cause it's there, you just gotta deal with it!

Alicia

Introduction

Alicia is sixteen. She is thin, with dark skin and a quiet voice. She spoke softly and tentatively and ended almost every statement with a soft, nervous laugh. In her first interview, Alicia said she was going to put the baby up for adoption as her mother wanted. During our first four interviews, Alicia talked about her pregnancy with this plan in mind.

She said her partner, Alexander, was eighteen and in the military. Alicia explained that when she got pregnant, it had been the first time she had had sex. During the pregnancy she had limited phone contact with Alex. He was not supportive of the plan to put the baby up for adoption.

While she was pregnant, Alicia lived with her aunt and attended an alternative high school. Alicia had phone contact with her mother, who lived out of state.

Over the course of our four interviews, Alicia seemed increasingly uncomfortable. She grew quieter and seemed hesitant to talk. When I asked her about this, she said she preferred not to think or talk about her situation and was just trying to let the time until delivery and adoption go by. At her request, we discontinued meeting.

We later met by chance and she said her situation had changed: Her mother had told her to keep the baby. I asked if she would be willing to meet for another interview. She agreed, and the material from our subsequent final interview will be presented separately after the material from the first interviews.

Narrative

First Four Interviews. I'm not very excited about being pregnant. I feel that I'm too young to take care of a baby. In terms of my age and finishing school. I'm sixteen and I found out when I was five months that I was pregnant. When I found out, it was kind of depressing. I thought I had ruined my life. I just wanted to get rid of it. When I went to get an abortion, they told me it was too late. They did a sonogram and I was already five months. It was too late, so I just have to deal with it. There's nothing I can do. I can't go in a back alley and take it out. So I try to look toward the best instead of looking down on myself. I'm just trying to live day-by-day. That's about it; I'm trying not to think too much about it.

I can't keep the baby. I have to give it up for adoption. I think it will be better for me that way because I have school to finish. That's what my mother wants me to do, so I think it'll be best. My mother made the decision for me. And I started thinking about it, she's right.

At first, when my mother found out I was pregnant, she wanted me to get an abortion, too. When I told her it was too late, she said that I had to give it up for adoption. My mother told me, "I'm not going to take care of no baby for you. You are too young. You'll wanna go out, you're not gonna watch that baby." I wasn't surprised when she said that. First of all, I can't imagine myself in this situation that I am in now.

When I got pregnant, it was the first time that I had ever had sex. The father of the baby, Alex, is in the military. He's eighteen; he travels a lot. I don't even know what he does, I try not to think about him. I knew him when I lived with my mother in Washington.

When I was with him, I thought that he was so responsible. I thought he would know better. But I was wrong. I told him to wear a condom. But he said no, that he'd take it out and I wouldn't get pregnant. I asked him about condoms, but he persuaded me into believing that he didn't need to wear one. He was like, "Come on, you can trust me." He just kept on talking a whole bunch of messages. It went into my head and I just believed him, like a fool. It was just his talking. That's all. He's the kind of person who says something and you just believe him.

After I found out I was pregnant, I called Alex because I thought he should know. When I first told him, he didn't know how to take it. I asked him, "What's wrong?" He said that he was scared but that he was happy in a way. But when I told him that my mother wanted me to give it up for adoption, he started cursing at me and stuff. So I just hung up on him. I haven't talked to him since.

When I found out that I couldn't have an abortion, at first, I sort of wanted to keep the baby. Before I got pregnant, every once in a while, I would think about having a baby. Just sometimes when I saw a cute little baby. But the reality, when you think about it, it's really hard. It ties you down. Not to be selfish, but I like to go out a lot. And I like quiet, I don't like to hear noisy babies crying. When I get older, I'll learn to deal with it—the noise and everything. It's just that I'm so young. I'm not even eighteen yet. I would think about having kids when I'm like twenty-seven, twenty-eight.

I used to look down on girls who used to get pregnant, especially the black females. That's what everybody expects from them, to have babies. It might not be true, but that's just how I felt. When you're out there you just pick that idea up from TV. And I learned it from my mother. It's kind of true. People think young black teenage girls are just out to get pregnant. Some of the time I can see what they are talking about. Especially the girls who have baby after baby after baby.

For instance, if you go to the county hospital, it seems like every Puerto Rican or black girl is pregnant or has a baby. My black female friends always ended up getting into trouble or pregnant, having kids or dropping out of school. Now I'm going to be another statistic or something like that. I didn't want to see myself like that.

The way my mother brought us up, we used to live in Washington. Where all the white people live, the rich part. There were a few black kids in my school, like four in my school. I was the only black kid achieving in school. So the black kids tried to put me down. They said I wanted to be with the white people because I was trying to make the same standards as the white kids. I guess they tried to put me down because they weren't achieving their goals. But I didn't really care, as long as I got my homework in on time.

My mother always made me feel good about that. My wanting to go to school and learn. She told me I could choose my goals. She knew I could achieve my goals regardless of who I was or where I went to school. My mother told me, "You got to do what you got to do, you can't let nobody hold you back." My mother told me, "If you think you're doing the right thing, just go out and do it."

My mother's the one who got me into modeling. That's what I'm doing for a career. Modeling was more my mother's interest than mine. She saw a modeling contest where you could win a thousand dollars for school. I wasn't too sure about it, but then after I won the contest, I was like "Maybe she was right." My mother said that she doesn't want me staying home taking care of a baby, because she wants me to do my modeling, to travel and stuff. I think I'll be better off doing that, too.

If the baby is with a good family, I would feel just as good as if it was with me. I do think about "Would I ever be able to see it in the future? Or should I just forget about it? Like it never happened?" I don't really know what to think about it.

Some people tell me that there was a reason why I got pregnant or they say, "God wanted you to get pregnant." I don't see no purpose in me getting pregnant at this age. If it would've happened later on in my life, it would have been different. But I think, "Why would God bless a teenage girl to take care of a little baby when she's not even taking care of herself?" I think about that when people tell me God wanted me to get pregnant. It makes no kind of sense whatsoever. I don't understand it myself.

Last Interview, After the Decision Not to Place the Baby for Adoption. My mother changed her mind, she decided I should keep it. She told me not to put the baby up for adoption. She said that if we put it up for adoption she would feel bad and she wouldn't be able to sleep at night if she knew the baby was with somebody else.

When she told me to keep it, I just said, "Oh, okay." I sort of knew it was going to come to that at the end. I'd had a feeling she'd change her mind since the beginning. And when she told me, I was happy. I don't know why. My aunt kept on telling me she was going to change her mind. So I was prepared for anything basically.

I don't think about any of that stuff that happened in the past. I'm not thinking about any of that adoption stuff. It's like it could have gone either way and it would have been for the best. I don't know. I can't explain it. If my mother told me to put it up for adoption, and I did, it would have been best. And if she told me to keep it, it would be best. I'm not going to say it didn't matter to me which way it went, but I try to think positive.

I just want to hurry up and get the pregnancy over with. I just want it to be over. Right now, I'm just waiting. I don't want nothing to go wrong. I'm not thinking too far ahead. There's no use thinking too much and when the time comes, something else ends up happening.

Besides me keeping it, I'm not sure what's going to happen now. I'll keep living with my aunt; she has her kids and she'll be there to help. And my mother is planning on moving back, too. I'm going to finish school since I only have one more year. I think that it will be difficult but I guess it depends on how the baby acts. If it's good and goes to sleep, I can get my homework done. But if it's always crying, I guess I can't get nothing accomplished. I'm trying not to think about it. We'll just see what happens. I'm not thinking too far ahead.

Alex, the father of the baby, called. He apologized and everything. He told me that he was sorry, that he should have been there. I just said, "All right, whatever." He said he wants to be there for me for the rest of the time, until I give birth to the baby. He says he'll send money but I don't need his money, he don't have to. If he wants to, he can, but if he don't, it don't matter. That's the way I feel—if he wants to be there, he can, but if he don't, he don't. I guess I just started disliking him for what he was doing. But I suppose I'll let him have some contact with the baby, I don't even know why. It's his, too, that's the only reason. But if it's a boy, I won't name it after him.

I'm hoping it'll be a girl. My mother said that if it was a girl she'd name it. I said okay, I'll let her name it. But if it is a boy, she said to name it after my father, since he had died. If it is a boy, I'll name it after my dad.

Tanya

Introduction

Tanya is a large young woman. She is seventeen, with light skin and a big voice. She was easily engaged in our first interview and spoke openly about her life. She was more guarded in talking about her partner, Kahleem, who she said was a small-time drug hustler. She seemed especially uncomfortable talking about the difference in their ages, that she was seventeen and he was twenty-seven. When I showed no negative reaction to this disclosure and inquired about why she thought I would have one, she seemed visibly relieved. When we ended, we agreed to meet again.

After she missed our appointment for a second interview, she came in to say that she had had a miscarriage. She said she would not be having further contact at the clinic since she planned to go away with her boyfriend. The following is from our only interview.

Narrative

Most of my friends have kids and some are already on their second child. Unfortunately, I was one of the last to become pregnant. I say unfortunately because it happened too soon. I wanted it to happen maybe after I was twenty-three. I wanted to go to school, finish school, and everything first. But, you know, it happens.

There's like ten of us that grew up together. And there's only one now who's not pregnant. I wanted to wait, but then after a while I just started feeling lonely. All my friends had kids and they basically want to do things with their children. They can't go to clubs; they can't go to parties.

They can't get baby-sitters. So it was like I would've had to get a whole set of new friends. But it's hard to find teenagers without kids.

Everybody I know is either pregnant or has a kid. Every time you turn around somebody's pregnant or they had a baby. You hear, "Did you hear such-and-such had a baby?" or "She's getting ready to go into labor any day now." I wonder when does it stop? Does anybody not have sex when they're teenagers?

Maybe it's because our hormones are crazy! Seems like everybody's just going out there and going for this. I don't know. Is it 'cause of single parents or is it tradition? Like when your mother has you young, she doesn't have much knowledge herself. And it continues—her daughter has a child young—the same situation I'm in. My mother had me when she was seventeen and I'm seventeen and having a baby. Actually, my great-grandmother had my grandmother when she was fourteen. And my grandmother had my mother at nineteen or eighteen.

What happened with me was I just got caught out there. Kahleem, my boyfriend, and I just went away for a vacation-type thing. It was kind of spur-of-the-moment and we just up and left with no pills, no nothing, nada. I had met him back in the summer when I was sixteen. And at the end of the summer, when I was supposed to go back to boarding school, we just decided he would come get me. So, I went to spend Labor Day weekend with him. The weekend came and passed and I said I was never going back to that school. That was the week I got pregnant.

Kahleem and I had talked about getting pregnant before, but we said we wanted to do it after we got married. We talked about how we wanted to have a baby after we bought a house, after we got everything established, so we'd have something to fall back on. We had thought about what if it happened now. But we was like, we ain't going to let that happen. Kahleem said if it did happen, that he'd be by my side. But I was thinking any guy's going to say that to make you feel good.

When I found out I was pregnant, I couldn't have an abortion. I don't believe in it. My family doesn't believe in it, put it that way. I was taught that when sperm and egg meet, that it's a life. So abortion was automatically scratched out of my mind.

My great-grandmother taught me that abortion is killing. She said, "You know what you're doing when you get involved. Don't use an abortion as contraception. That's killing." She would say, "There is contraception, so why don't you use it? You could take only two seconds and put a condom on, what's the problem? Or you take the pill, keep it up every day, what's the problem? It's you. You people are careless, foolish, deal with it." So, that's what I'm doing.

That cycle of having babies young has to stop. I don't want my child to be pregnant as a teenager. I don't. I really want to stress that. If I have to lock her up or lock him up, I'm going to. I don't want them getting pregnant young. I'm gonna tell them not to, and tell them that it's very hard. It's hard because being pregnant has caused a lot of resentment from my family. I don't even speak to them.

I think the thing about tradition and mothers having babies young is, instead of your mother trying to be your mother, she wants to be your friend. Instead of taking discipline where it's supposed to be, your mother wants to be buddy-buddy. I don't know how to explain it. It's like your mother wants to do everything with you and be on a teenage level. She doesn't encourage you to have sex, but she's like "If you go ahead and do it, it's all right, I don't care." She'd say, "I understand why you do it" or "I understand why you do drugs and all. But if you want help I'll get you help if you want it." I felt like "Well, what kind of discipline are you giving me? What kind of role model are you?" I wanted to tell my mother, "You're not a role model for me." That's why, whenever I needed anything, I went to my great-grandmother.

My great-grandmother raised me. She taught me my morals and values and everything. God bless her, though, she's dead now. She's been dead for three years, but she gave me my background. She gave me my backbone, to be the woman I am today. She taught me to stand up for what I believe in and to do the right thing.

I lived with my great-grandmother since I was born. The reason why I was so close to her was because she was on her deathbed when I was born. When I was only a week old, they left me in the room with her. The family was out in the living room and she was in a back room and they heard me crying, screaming. My grandmother said, "Just leave her in there" to see what my great-grandmother would do. My great-grandmother got the energy and strength to pick me up and calm me down and ever since no one ever took me away from her. And she lived for another thirteen years after that. So everybody called me her "miracle baby."

I was never close with my mother. I was always with my great-grandmother; my mother went her way, I went mine. Anyway, I never really considered her my mother. I don't look like my mother and so a lot of people didn't believe that she was my mother.

It didn't bother me that I didn't look like my mother. I was light like my great-grandmother. My mother was darker than me. She wasn't that dark, but she was like an Indian complexion. I am the lightest thing in my family. That doesn't bother me. Other people look at it funny that I'm so light. But I feel like my skin color's none of their business. I think that a human being is only a human being. 'Cause if you take everybody's skin off, we all have red blood. Word up.

One time there was this racial thing in my school, when I was in boarding school in Pennsylvania and people started fighting. They said, "Well, the blacks on one side and the whites on the other side." And then, they said, "Well, Tanya, what side do you go on?" So I said, "I'm on my own side. I don't care what you all do, kill each other, whatever, but I'm the one who will be still living and getting my education."

I had to go to boarding school because my grandmother sent me there. She made me take a test and I got a scholarship to go. I didn't know what the test was for at the time. If I knew what it was for, I would have failed it on purpose. I was twelve when my grandmother shipped me off; that was the year before my great-grandmother died. I hated my grandmother for sending me away then because I felt I needed to be with my great-grandmother all the time.

Since my great-grandmother died, I've basically been on my own. No one can ever replace her. I won't allow no one to get close to me like that ever again. It'll never happen. That's a part of me that I don't want to be touched. And right now, the only one I have is Kahleem. He did a lot for me, he's stood by my side and everything. I wasn't sure what he'd do, but he stood up and did the right thing. His support means a lot to me. I really need it. Without him, I don't know what I'd do.

3

Desire and Denial

Their Pregnancies

It Happened/I Wanted It

A theme that emerged for all of the participants about pregnancy was "It happened." This seemed to indicate that they felt that pregnancy was something that had occurred that was out of their control; Alicia's situation clearly fits this. Five of the six participants expressed two concepts simultaneously—"It happened" and "I wanted it." The latter concept seemed to suggest something sought and potentially within their control. Thus, the young women seemed to maintain dual, potentially conflicting, perspectives on the event.

In their assessments about the occurrence of their pregnancies, the participants may be seen on a continuum. At one end is Alicia, who felt strongly that her pregnancy just happened; at the other end is Chantel, who expressed having sought to become pregnant.

In discussing their pregnancies, five of the six participants said they wouldn't have thought they would be pregnant at this age. They reported that this was not what others, nor what they themselves, might previously have expected. Although this represented a shift, most seemed accepting of this change in plans. Most noted an awareness of peers, friends, or family who as adolescents had had children.

Alicia will be described first; then the group of Kim, Shamika, Tanya, Edouine, and Chantel will be addressed. Alicia described the circumstances of her pregnancy as happenstance; it was the first time she had had sex. She attributed the occurrence to her partner's persuasiveness, her own gullibility, and chance. Alicia reported that she had had no intention of becoming pregnant at this age. She said, "I can't imagine myself in the situation that I'm in now."

Alicia stated her awareness of stereotypes of black teenage girls with babies and the conflict her situation engendered. She said, "My black female friends always ended up getting into trouble or pregnant, having kids or dropping out of school. Now I'm going to be another statistic or something like that. I didn't want to see myself like that." In discussing her pregnancy, Alicia struggled to incorporate an event that was neither planned nor wanted; she said that she saw "no purpose" to her becoming pregnant at this age. She was depending on her mother to tell her what to do about the pregnancy.

Kim, Tanya, and Shamika each said about their pregnancy, "It happened," and at the same time expressed mixed feelings about having wanted to get pregnant. Kim said that she had thought a lot about pregnancy. She was quick to say that although she wasn't deliberately trying to get pregnant, the issue of pregnancy was always present. Kim said, "I mean it's not like I set out to try to get pregnant, but whenever I'd have sex, I'd think, 'What's going to happen with us? What if I got pregnant?' And with Colin, I thought it was different." Although she couldn't explain this further, she attributed her wanting to get pregnant to having had strong feelings for Colin. Kim's perspective on her pregnancy was that it was something that had happened that she wanted.

Kim said that people she went to school with were surprised that she was pregnant. She expressed the view that getting pregnant at this age also contradicted her own previous ideas about pregnancy. Kim said, "When I was fifteen, I would get really scared about possibly being pregnant." She said that this was because she had been following her mother's plan for her life: to pursue "school, college, marriage, and then kids." Kim said that her current plans for the future still incorporated these events but in a different order.

Kim described her relationship with a close friend who had decided to maintain her pregnancy and was now a single parent. Kim compared her own situation to her friend's.

Tanya presented her pregnancy in relation to her peers. She said that most of her friends had children and were even "on their second child," and that she was one of the last to become pregnant. Tanya described the occurrence of her pregnancy as something that "just happened." She said that the pregnancy occurred when she and Kahleem were away on vacation. However, the circumstances and timing of her having discontinued her birth control pills were somewhat unclear.

Although Tanya reported that she had wanted to get pregnant, she said that her pregnancy went against her previously held belief of the need to wait to have children. Tanya described, "I wanted it to happen maybe after I was twenty-three. I wanted to go to school, finish school and everything." Tanya said that she used to talk to others about the importance of postponing childbearing and that her current situation presented her with a conflict. Tanya explained that although pregnancy made her feel as if she was "being a hypocrite," it happened and she must deal with it.

Shamika said that she had been very surprised to learn she was pregnant, that pregnancy had "just happened." Shamika described her current pregnancy in relation to her experience of an abortion. Following that experience, which left her sad and angry, she said she had decided that if she ever got pregnant again, she would maintain the pregnancy.

Shamika described having had mixed feelings after that experience and said that this pregnancy had happened in spite of using contraception. She reported that she had been taking birth control pills, though inconsistently. When Shamika evaluated the possibility that Jamal might have intended to get her pregnant, she said that because they didn't necessarily know she was going to get pregnant at that particular time, it "just happened."

Shamika discussed the fact that several of her friends had children, although she did not relate this to her own pregnancy. She did not suggest having thought that she would wait to get pregnant, nor did she feel that having a baby would be much of a change.

The other two participants, Edouine and Chantel, spoke about how they had wanted and were trying to get pregnant when "it happened." Edouine presented a mixed assessment of the occurrence of her pregnancy. She said that she hadn't used condoms with Khary because she wanted to have his child. Although pregnancy was desired and sought, Edouine also felt that the pregnancy had happened. She described that "it wasn't like we were trying to have a baby but we said, 'If it happens, it happens.'"

Edouine also said that her pregnancy went against a previously held belief about waiting until she was older to have children. Edouine said, "I always wanted to have kids . . . but I never thought I would have it at this young age." She commented on the fact that she felt her mother wouldn't be too upset about the pregnancy since her mother had had her first child when she was fifteen. Edouine also noted her older sister's experience as a single parent.

Chantel said that although she had planned and sought pregnancy with Stephen, she was nevertheless surprised when it happened. She reported that she had calculated when she was ovulating and that they had been having unprotected sex on those days. Although they were seeking pregnancy, she was surprised when she got pregnant. She said, "For some odd reason, I just didn't think that it was going to happen."

Chantel described how getting pregnant at this age contradicted her previous ideas about waiting to have a child. She said: "I guess the time to get pregnant would be like twenty, twenty-one, twenty-two. Something like that. Everybody's like, finish school first, get a good job. I felt like that, too, but it happened."

Chantel said that although she had wanted to wait, she had sought pregnancy. She explained that while she was in the group home, she had seen other girls with babies who made her think about having one. She said, "They made it look so nice. So lovey-dovey." She described that she felt a baby would offer her love. Although she was unsure about her plans for the future, Chantel said she felt that her plans would subsequently become clearer.

Life Is Hard; This Baby Will Give Me Something I Need

This theme held for Kim, Edouine, and Chantel. All three expressed the perspective that their lives had been difficult; however, they were unsentimental in sharing this assessment. Rather, by talking about their early circumstances, they seemed to provide the context or rationale for their decisions and actions. Each expressed the idea that she had had to grow up fast and had learned that she had to take care of herself. As a result, these participants felt they had to take responsibility for getting what they wanted. Each one, although stating a different reason, said that she believed a baby would provide something she needed. They presented the perspective that a baby was something they desired because it would fulfill a need.

Kim felt the baby would provide her a sense of responsibility and a new life. Kim said that her life had been difficult. She explained, "It was very stressful. Nothing about my life was very normal." Kim assessed, "There were things that made me grow up earlier." These factors included having had an older father and a strict mother, being Chinese and black, and being teased for looking like a boy.

Kim said these influences had contributed to her being "messed up." She said that she tended toward depression; she presented her reasons for wanting a baby in this context. She explained that she often relied on other people to pull her out of her depression. She said, "That's why I'm using this baby; to pull myself up." To Kim, the baby was a new life, *her* new life of "doing things and taking responsibility." The baby seemed to provide her with a sense of optimism and initiative. It seemed that she planned to do things for the baby that she felt she could not have done for herself.

Edouine discussed her pregnancy in the context of lessons she had learned about life. Edouine explained that dealing with her alcoholic mother had taught her that she was on her own. She said, "When I was thirteen, I just realized I have to take care of myself." She felt that whatever she wanted, she must get for herself; she explained, "I've got to look out for my own self."

Edouine's pregnancy fit with this perspective in that she has to do what she has to do for herself. She presented her pregnancy as something she wanted. Although she later described how her feelings had shifted, she said that she had always wanted a child and that she had sought to have a baby with Khary.

Like Kim, Edouine said that she had had to grow up quickly. Edouine noted that due to her life experiences, she was wise beyond her years and people often didn't believe that she was only sixteen.

Chantel also expressed the perspective that she had been damaged by the events in her life. She said that she felt "emotionally shot from all the things that have happened" in her life. Chantel said that when she was fifteen, she had realized that she had to take care of herself. She described how this caused a shift in her perspective. She said, "I was thinking about it, and I realized it is all about me. You have to do what you have to do for yourself, what's best for you. Forget about everybody else. So I started thinking about self, self, self." For Chantel, this involved a sense of having to do things for herself and a responsibility to take control. She elaborated, "I feel like you only live once, say what you have to say, do what you have to do."

Chantel connected her history of rejection to her reasons for having a child. She believed a baby would provide something she needed and had lacked. Chantel explained that most of her life she had been rejected. She said that she always wanted somebody to love her; she had always wanted to be loved. Chantel said that her parents had judged and rejected her and the baby represented the opportunity to get something different. Chantel said, "The baby will accept me for who and what I am. . . . I know I can't be rejected by this child because this is my child."

This theme did not apply to Shamika, Alicia, and Tanya. Neither Shamika nor Alicia presented awareness that their lives had been difficult, nor did they suggest that their pregnancy had a purpose or would fulfill a need. They both presented the perspective that the pregnancy just happened due to circumstances. Alicia in particular struggled to deal with her assessment that there was no purpose to her being pregnant. Although Tanya's description of her life included her view that her life had been difficult, in our one interview she did not suggest any related purpose or need to her pregnancy.

Deal with It!

This theme held for five of the six participants. All except Edouine used this phrase in talking about their pregnancies. The phrase seemed to connote acceptance or an attitude of pragmatism and inevitability as a response to pregnancy. The participants' comments suggested they believed that some things must be accepted without option. For some participants—Tanya and Chantel—pregnancy was seen as a necessary consequence. For the others, it seemed that this was just how it must be. The statement "Deal with it," especially as expressed by Shamika and Alicia, also seemed to minimize any emotional reaction to the event.

The five here described their situations with resignation and pragmatism. These participants presented a philosophy that they just had to cope with their difficult circumstances. Kim assessed, "The relationship itself took a good few months out of my life. It's going to end up taking eighteen years out of my life, actually more like the rest of my life. I'm dealing with it." In talking about the future, Kim expressed a similar attitude. When she talked about her fears related to pregnancy, she said, "I hope nothing bad will come out of it. If something does, though, I will deal with it."

Shamika's description of her reaction to learning she was pregnant included pragmatic acceptance. She said, "At first I was a little surprised, then I just had to deal with it." This also applied to her fears about the future; she said, "I don't listen to what other people say about being a mother. Everybody's different. I just don't ask them. I'd just rather see for myself. If I made the biggest mistake of my life, I have to deal with it. . . . I chose it so I will just have to deal with it." When asked to identify what the most important thing was about pregnancy for her, Shamika responded, "Deal with it!" When asked what that meant, Shamika said, "It's too late now. 'Cause it's there, you might as well deal with it."

Alicia's strategy of coping with her pregnancy also involved a pragmatic attitude. She said, "I have to deal with it, so I look for the better, look toward the best for myself rather than looking down on myself." She revealed a similar pragmatism in her reaction to learning she was pregnant. She said, "When I went to get an abortion, they told me it was too late. . . . It was too late, so I just have to deal with it. There's nothing I can do. I can't go in a back alley and take it out."

When asked how she felt about not being able to have an abortion, Alicia said, "Well, no kind of specific way really. I just have to deal with it." Alicia explained how she was managing her pregnancy: "I'm just dealing. I just try to live day-by-day. Just go to school, do my work. I'm just waiting for it to be through. Trying not to feel." When asked what would happen if she let herself feel, she said, "Nothing. I just don't."

Tanya expressed a philosophy of "Deal with it" in accepting her pregnancy. She explained how she told Kahleem that she was pregnant and that she wouldn't have an abortion or put the baby up for adoption. She said that she told him, "It's going to be mine, and I'm going to deal with it." Tanya said that her great-grandmother had taught her that if one was foolish about birth control, one must deal with the consequences.

Chantel presented a similarly pragmatic philosophy about dealing with pregnancy as a consequence. She said, "If you're responsible enough to have sex, then you're responsible enough to take care of the baby. You are responsible enough to deal with the consequences. The consequences is a baby! . . . I felt that way after I got pregnant. This is it, you know. Paying the consequences."

Once You're Pregnant, You Have to Think About the Future/I'm Just Living Day-to-Day

Four of the six participants said that being pregnant necessitated thoughts about the future. They presented this as a shift in their thinking. Most of these participants discussed this development in relation to their plans about school. In talking about the future, these participants also raised concerns about money, child care, and the stresses of parenting. In Kim's case, this was most explicit, whereas in Shamika's, this was only hinted at ("If I made the worst mistake of my life, I will just have to deal with it").

Although these participants stressed the importance of thinking about the future, at the same time they also used the phrase "I'm living day-to-day." This seemed to mean that there are things they "can't plan" (Kim, Alicia, Edouine), or "can't know" (Shamika), ahead of time. This seemed to be a pragmatic attitude that helped them to cope with their uncertainty and worry about the future. In some instances, the participants seemed to deny that the future would be difficult (Chantel, Shamika) and, in others, to present hopeful fantasies about it (Kim, Edouine, and Chantel).

In discussing their futures, three of these participants (Kim, Chantel, and Edouine) mentioned hopes for their children. They each said that they wanted their children to have different and better lives than they had had.

Kim explained that following pregnancy she thought more about the future. She described, "Once you have a baby you start wondering about the future. You start making plans and trying to be more responsible." She elaborated, "The reason it wasn't clear was because it wasn't my path. Those were my mother's plans for me, not mine. So how could I fill in the details? Now that I'm pregnant, I know what I want to do, I actually know what career I want."

She said she had had doubts about her abilities but her pregnancy necessitated change. This was due to her increased responsibility for a baby. Kim explained, "Before, I could have said that I wouldn't need to eat for a week, but I can't say that now. I can't say that my baby will go without diapers for a while. There are things I have to do for the baby."

Kim said that she worried about finances, supplies, and how she would attend college. She said uncertainty about the future was difficult. She explained, "It's hard. I worry a lot. I worry about what's going to happen. I just want to know if I can do it, how it's going to be." Kim's ideas about the future included wanting her child to have a good life. She described that she wanted to do things differently from the way she was raised.

Shamika discussed the future in terms of a belief in the importance of school. She said, "I know you can't do nothing without an education, so I'm going to go to school." Like Kim, Shamika noted a shift in her perspective following pregnancy. She asserted, "I have to really get serious in school now." She noted, "Before it used to be hard to go to school. But once you're pregnant you just gotta think about things. That's what you do. I can't mess up in school because what kind of life will I have for the baby if I don't have a high school diploma? You have to ask yourself those questions."

Shamika expressed two conflicting perspectives about her future. On one hand, she said that she had thought about the possibility that she might have made "the biggest mistake" of her life. On the other, she said she felt that nothing would be different following having the baby.

Edouine said that she planned to finish school because of her pregnancy. Edouine said it was important to get an education so that the child wouldn't respond, "But you didn't get one," when she told him or her to go to school. She described her plans following the baby: "I'll finish school, go like to a year in college, get pregnant, and after the baby is like three years old in nursery school or whatever, go back to work, and have a morning or like a day job. And at night, have my child and have a nice house, apartment."

She expressed worries about money, the possibility of not having the baby's father's support, and of not finishing school or having a stable place to live. However, she said she coped with these through different strategies: "It's hard now, and I haven't even had the baby. I don't want to get myself in a state of depression, so I've got to do something. I go outside or something. I don't want to get myself all worked up on crying over nothing. It's not going to help."

In talking about the future, Edouine spoke of her hopes for her child: "I want them to be different than I was in a lot of ways. Because my life was terrible." She also expressed hopes regarding her child's education: "I don't want my kid to be raised up the way I was raised up or to drop out of school like I did and to do something easier like to go get a GED. I want my child to stay in school."

Like the others, Chantel stressed the importance of school in relation to having a child: "I think that's a necessity. I mean, how are you going to help your child in school if you didn't go to school." Although she was not sure about her current direction, she said her pregnancy presented an opportunity to plan for the future.

Chantel explained, "I thought I knew what I wanted to do at one time. Because I went to college for a year. But now I believe that's not really what I want to do. So, now being pregnant, I can think about what I want to do." She added, "Now I have an excuse to be out of school and think about what I want to do."

Chantel said that she didn't feel the future with a baby would be that different. She explained that since she was currently staying up practically all night being pregnant, "I don't think the staying up with the baby will be hard." However, she alluded to an awareness of the difficulties of continuing school with the baby. She then described her image of how things would be different for her child than they were for her. She said, "I will struggle for my child, I will struggle if I have to. But my child will never know that we're struggling because he or she will be content. I will do everything to make my child happy."

Although Alicia described some plans for the future, she said she was currently living day-to-day. This was especially true early in her pregnancy when she was planning to put the baby up for adoption. Even after she had decided to keep the baby, she did not discuss much about the pregnancy in relation to her thoughts of the future. Although she seemed to minimize her worries, the ones she did disclose revealed that she had serious concerns.

Alicia said, "I'm just wishing days would go quick. I just try to live day-by-day. I'm just waiting for it to be through. Trying not to feel." When asked about the future, Alicia responded, "I don't know what it will be like after I have the baby. I have to wait and see, I don't know." She continued, "People have different feelings. I hear different stories, so I really don't know. I hear after delivery, some people go into depression and a whole bunch of weird stuff. I don't know. I hope I don't; I don't like being sad."

Her ideas about continuing school included an awareness of the difficulties of doing this with a child. Alicia said, "I'm going to finish school since I only have one more year. I think that it will be difficult but I guess it depends on how the baby acts. If it's good and goes to sleep, I can get my homework done. But if it's always crying, I guess I can't get nothing accomplished."

Tanya did not express the theme that pregnancy prompted her to think about the future. This may be due to the fact that we had only one interview.

Reflections on the Themes About Pregnancy

Of the four themes about pregnancy, the theme "It happened/I wanted it" is primary because it embraces what seemed to be a contradiction at the heart of the participants' views of their pregnancies. When participants first said, "It happened," I thought they just weren't admitting a more conscious desire and action to get pregnant. This was Dash's (1989) experience in conducting ethnographic research with a similar population. I initially expected that with enough rapport these participants could trust me with a similar revelation. This seemed to be confirmed by my experience with Edouine, who, after encouragement that she wouldn't be judged, said, "To tell you the honest truth, I wanted to have [Khary's] child." However, in the next breath, she restated that the pregnancy "just happened." This was the case with my other participants; the finding was clearly more complex.

The seeming contradiction of this theme may suggest the participants' ambivalence and ambiguity about the occurrence of their pregnancies. Adler and Tschann (1993), for example, found that there is more motivation for pregnancy than is generally acknowledged at a "preconscious" level. At this level, pregnancy is seen as desirable although not actively sought. Although perspectives such as this provide an additional way of looking at adolescent pregnancy, they do little to increase our understanding or to engage the complexity of meanings within the participants' social context. It seems more important to approach understanding in a way that considers the meanings from the participants' perspectives.

One possibility is that the duality "It happened/I wanted it" may reflect that the participants do not want to assert an unambiguous desire for, or control over, pregnancy. Their comments suggest that pregnancy and parenthood represent a big undertaking about which they have fears and concerns. Perhaps by saying and believing "It happened" the participants are protecting themselves from confronting the responsibility and reality of such an action. Such use of language to create and structure reality has been addressed within postmodernist thought.[1]

Other possible explanations for the seeming contradiction of this theme address the fact that the participants expressed a disbelieving attitude toward the occurrence of pregnancy. This was true even for those who had actively sought pregnancy; as Chantel said, "For some odd reason, I didn't think it would happen." This is consistent with literature on adolescents' cognitive development and adolescents' beliefs about invulnerability.[2]

That all of the participants described their pregnancy with "It happened" is consistent with much of the literature on attribution or locus of control. According to this perspective, the participants might be seen as having high external loci of control. This suggests they believed that reinforcing events occurred independently of their actions and that the future is determined more by chance and luck.

The idea that lower-SES black people tend to attribute causation as being outside their control has been forwarded by some as an element of black psychology (Franklin, 1987). However, this concept has often been applied pejoratively to black people (Banks, Ward, McQuater, & DeBritto, 1991). Others from cross-cultural perspectives, including Sue and Sue (1990), have countered with concepts that acknowledge that worldviews differ among populations.

Sue and Sue (1990) have suggested that different social and cultural experiences need to be taken into account in making assessments about locus of control. They argued that the worldviews of "minority populations" may differ from those of the "dominant culture." They suggested that these worldviews are influential because they "affect how we think, make decisions, behave, and define events" (p. 137).

Sue and Sue also asserted the importance of locus of responsibility in the formation of life orientations. *Locus of responsibility* refers to the degree of blame placed on the individual or system. Individuals' orientations tend to be either person-centered or situation/system-centered. People with a situation- or system-centered orientation view the sociocultural environment as more potent than an individual's influence.

Sue and Sue (1990) emphasized the role that racism and the subordinate position assigned to minorities in society play in the development of worldviews. The participants' statements that pregnancy "happened" suggest that they may believe less in their agency to determine their own fate and that they place less responsibility on themselves for what has transpired and more on the situation. These may be seen as part of a worldview developed within their particular sociocultural context. The participants' experiences of racial discrimination, the influence of racism on identity development, and expectations and realities related to achievement must be noted. In sum, Sue and Sue's (1990) work supports the importance of considering the participants' worldviews and their sociocultural contexts as these relate to pregnancy.

Such a consideration entails addressing several related beliefs about life. The first of these beliefs is that, in the participants' views, many things happen to them and are out of their control. This was especially true for Chantel and Edouine; their descriptions of life featured uncertainty about who or what they could count on. Given the participants' experiences and contexts, it seems difficult or unwise to plan or to assert any deliberate control. Their statements that pregnancy "happened" seem to reflect this reality.

A second, related belief is that of self-reliance. The participants said they had learned early that they are on their own despite some involvement by others. Their comments suggest that they have not been able to depend on authority figures in their lives. The participants said they believed they must get what they need for themselves. These beliefs, and their relationship to the participants' pregnancies, are contained in the theme "Life is hard; this baby will give me something I need." Kim, Edouine, and Chantel described themselves as having experienced difficult circumstances that influenced who they are and how they do things. They connected these experiences to their reasons for having a baby.

The participants' perspectives that "life is hard" also relates to a sense of maturity. Their reflections contained assessments that they felt they were forced to grow up quickly and had experienced more than their years would suggest.

It has been suggested that poor black children are not often granted the luxury of childhood or adolescence (Elise, 1995; Ladner, 1971). Given that reality, it seems that it may be a more normative possibility to have a baby at a younger age. Social constructionist perspectives of adolescence, such as Taylor's (1994), suggest the importance of assessing cultural differences in determining the meaning of *adolescence*.

In considering the meanings of the themes about pregnancy, it is important to note that all of the participants mentioned friends or relatives who, as adolescents, had had babies. Within their contexts, they had peers with children. As Tanya noted, "Most of my friends have kids and some are already on their second child. . . . There's like ten of us that grew up together. And there's only one now who's not pregnant." It seems that, for some, becoming pregnant was normative among their peer group.

It is also important that when "it happened," they got pregnant—they were in a relationship. This will be addressed in depth in Chapter 5 about themes related to the babies' fathers. However, it is relevant to note here that the participants identified that their relationships with the babies' fathers had offered them something they wanted. This included the possibility of love and a positive relationship. These seemed especially important given their histories and circumstances. The possibility of other "rewards" or advantages to having a baby are expressed by the theme "This baby will give me something I need." These rewards include a sense of independence and the chance to redo or correct one's own life experience.

The seeming contradiction of the theme "It happened/I wanted it" may also reflect the participants' awareness of a norm of not saying that they wanted to get pregnant at this age. All of the participants said that they had previously believed and espoused the idea that they should wait to have children. Kim's comments illustrate the "ideal norm"; she said she was taught that "you go to school, get a job, then you get married and have children."

Each of the participants said that she would not have expected to be pregnant at this age. They said that although they had thought about the possibility of pregnancy, they believed that it was something that would happen later, after they finished school. Tanya's statements exemplify this perspective. She said, "I wanted it to happen maybe after I was twenty-three. I wanted to go to school, finish school, and everything first. But, you know, it happens."

It seemed the "ideal" norm of waiting to have a baby may have been at variance with their desires to have a baby, their beliefs about life, and an awareness of an "actual" norm they saw enacted by peers who as adolescents have had babies. Although the participants had been told that having a baby would hinder their chances at success, they see a different reality around them. Given the fact that they feel they have to take responsibility for what they get in life, they may take that chance, especially given their hopes to fulfill their needs. Their beliefs also suggest that having a baby may seem like a reasonable choice. Given this context, a baby seems to be something the young woman wants and needs; she must act for herself in creating her life.

As a related issue, several of the participants said that at the time they got pregnant, they had been uncertain about their plans for the future. It seemed they had lost their direction in school. Kim, Edouine, Shamika, and Tanya said that at that time they hadn't been doing well, or had disliked school, and had not wanted to continue. Similarly, Chantel said that she was unsure about her career goals after having started college. This lack of direction might be related to the fact that pregnancy "happened." Due to uncertainty about their plans for the future, they may have lacked the incentive they had previously had to prevent pregnancy. Recent research suggests that, contrary to traditional assumptions that young women have children and drop out of school, many adolescent mothers are in the process of "dropping out" when they become pregnant (Luker, 1996). This supports the perspective that adolescents need reasons to delay parenthood.[3]

In discussing their pregnancies, participants suggested that pregnancy meant they had to "get serious about school." It seemed that pregnancy offered a reason to recommit to their education, perhaps to achieve for their children what they couldn't do for themselves. It seemed that internal motivation to attend school may have been difficult to maintain. Research on teen pregnancy and high school completion suggests that teen mothers' sense of responsibility to their children contributes to their commitment to education (Jacobs, 1994; Elise, 1995).

The themes about pregnancy embrace a variety of complex issues; these include the participants' beliefs about life, the future, their partners, and themselves. The seeming contradiction of the central theme, "It happened/I wanted it," may reflect their conflict and ambivalence about these issues. In particular, it may reflect conflict between the norms of the "ideal" they have been taught and the "real" they experience.

This is supported by Ladner's (1971) work that explored the process of becoming a woman within a lower-income black community. About the young women she studied, Ladner said, "In a sense they are caught between two worlds—the Black community and the larger society" (p. 178). They are also caught between two community prescriptions of behavior: "To have a child represents fulfillment of the womanly tradition in the Black community and, as such, is not viewed entirely in the realm of stigmatization" (p. 217).

The participants' comments suggest that they experience some conflict between these two norms that may affect their own self-perceptions. They seem acutely aware of others' and, often, their own previous judgments about teenagers, especially black teens, having babies.[4] The participants seemed to struggle to incorporate the fact that they are pregnant in light of these beliefs; as Tanya said, "I feel like I'm a hypocrite." This finding suggests the implications of being caught between these norms for their self-image and esteem. The participants' difficulties in accommodating the change and in managing the potential conflict between the two norms may also be reflected in the seeming contradiction of "It happened/I wanted it."

That the participants negotiate these issues with a certain practicality is suggested by the theme "Deal with it!" This straightforward attitude toward pregnancy may reflect an ethic of pragmatism identified among black Americans (Gwaltney, 1980; White, 1984). In White's (1984) treatment of black psychology, he suggested, "The first step of learning to survive is to see life exactly as it is without self-deception or romantic pieties" (p. 29). Although the participants acknowledged the possible severity of the situation following delivery, they said they could only wait to see what would happen. As Shamika said, "If I made the biggest mistake of my life, I have to deal with it." Given their circumstances, it seemed this could be a more reasonable risk than might have been imagined.

Notes

1. See Riger (1992).
2. See Franklin (1987) and Morrison (1985).
3. Gibbs (1992) and Scott-Jones et al. (1989).
4. This is consistent with Kaplan's (1997) findings.

4

Abandonment and Difference

Their Mothers' Influence

My Mother Wasn't There for Me

This theme was true for four of the six participants in that their discussions featured the lack or loss of their mothers. Edouine, Tanya, and Chantel had been left by their mothers at birth and had had limited, often negative, contact with their mothers. Another participant, Kim, described that although her mother had been physically present, Kim had felt abandoned by her emotionally.

These participants were candid in discussing their mothers' unavailability or loss. Their comments also suggested an awareness of difficulties in the mothers' lives and some acceptance or forgiveness because of this. Nevertheless, the participants seemed to struggle to understand their mothers' feelings and actions. The participants expressed feelings of abandonment, rejection, and loss; their comments revealed resignation, anger, disappointment, and confusion.

The four discussed here expressed the perspective that their mothers hadn't been there for them. Edouine indicated that she was aware that she had not gotten what she needed from her mother. In discussing her perspective, Edouine presented some understanding of her mother's disease. Edouine explained, "When she drinks she just don't care about nobody but herself and her alcoholism." Edouine said that, as a result, she had learned to take care of herself and to do things for herself.

In spite of her experiences of disappointment and abandonment, Edouine didn't thoroughly reject her mother. Rather, she seemed to accept her mother within the limits of her availability. Edouine asserted, "I would like my mother to be there, but I can't really depend on my mother. My mother is important to me, but my mother is not stable."

In describing her situation, Tanya explained that because her mother was addicted to drugs Tanya had been raised from birth by her great-grandmother. Tanya summarized her belief about her mother's attitude when she left her with the great-grandmother. She said, "So my mother she just felt like 'Well, that's a burden off me.' She could do whatever she wanted to do, so she did."

Tanya questioned her mother's actions. Tanya suggested her mother's actions might relate to the fact that she was a teenage mother. In describing her feelings about her mother, Tanya expressed anger that her mother had provided her with neither discipline nor an example. Tanya said that she had wanted her mother to be a role model, not a friend. Tanya described, "When my mother did that, it really irked me a lot because I wanted a mother. I didn't want a friend. I can get a friend in the streets. That's why I didn't always turn to my mother. She was too much on a friendship level; she couldn't be a mother to me."

Chantel's descriptions of her life featured an acute awareness of rejection: by her birth mother, her biological father, and her foster mother. Of these rejections, it seemed Chantel struggled most to understand her biological mother's actions and to accept them in light of her mother's mental illness. Chantel said, "My mother and father just sent me away. . . . My mother, she had the problem. She's mentally ill or whatever. That's another thing I don't understand. If you're mentally ill, why have a child? But anyway, I don't know, I wasn't there."

These rejections had influenced her greatly; she said that they were the reason she wanted a baby. Chantel felt that a baby would give her love. It would neither judge nor reject her. Even as she pursued her remedy for these rejections, Chantel still struggled to understand her parents' actions. She questioned whether she might be responsible in some way and questioned her parents' reasoning. Chantel continued, "I can't tell you what they judged me for, my father and my mother. I know they didn't want me."

Kim's situation was somewhat different in that Kim described her mother as being physically present and strict in Kim's upbringing. However, Kim said that her mother was Chinese and had rejected Kim because she was black. Kim described that her mother had been emotionally absent. Kim said, "She was there, but she wasn't there emotionally." She explained that "when I had a lot of problems, she just didn't understand. . . . She couldn't understand." Kim had wanted her mother to give her emotional support and love. Kim said that she struggled to understand why her mother hadn't provided these. She attributed this lack to their differences in age, race, and culture.

Kim maintained a relationship with her mother and said that she would still like her mother's support. However, as a result of disappointment, Kim said she had lowered her expectations of her mother. About wanting her mother's support, Kim said, "You can't plan what another person is going to do. . . . That's why I'm not planning on what my mother may or may not do. If it happens, it will make my life easier."

This theme did not hold true for Alicia and Shamika. Both said that they had relatively close relationships with their mothers and, until recently, had lived with their mothers. In contrast to the other participants' reports of their mothers, Alicia's and Shamika's descriptions of their mothers were fairly positive. Both described their mothers as having gainful employment, stable relationships with men, and active involvement in the daughters' lives.

I'm Not like My Mother

Four of the six participants expressed sentiments of not being like, and not wanting to be like, their mothers. Three of these—Kim, Edouine, and Chantel—were those who voiced the theme "My mother wasn't there for me." Kim expressed the theme of not being like her mother most clearly. Her actions and philosophy are those of rebellion against her mother's wishes and values. Edouine was also explicit in describing how she has lived life defining herself as different from her mother. Chantel and Alicia expressed that they wanted to be different from their mothers in certain areas of their lives.

These participants' comments suggest that they have used their mothers in defining their own identities. As they asserted that they were different, and had sought this difference, they simultaneously acknowledged their mothers' influence. Questions about the possible similarities between themselves and their mothers ran throughout their discussions.

The four here—Kim, Edouine, Chantel, and Alicia—expressed the belief that they were different from their mothers. Kim's lifestyle, actions, and decisions revolved around rebelling against her mother. She described herself as different from her mother and tried to separate from her through rebellion. Kim's assessment that she was different from her mother included differences in age, cultural upbringing, values, and experience. In describing her life, Kim identified her mother as a pivotal influence. Kim said, "I had to rebel a lot because I never really got to do anything I wanted to do. My mother was so strict and controlling that I used to rebel. I started having a life, a social life, and having a sexual life that she didn't know about."

Kim viewed her actions in light of these motives. She seems connected to her mother in rebellion; she framed her decision to maintain her pregnancy within this context. Kim said, "I guess I should've waited until I'd made up my mind about what I was going to do before telling my mother so she wouldn't influence me."

Kim explained that although she had been leaning toward having an abortion, her mother's actions pushed her the opposite way. Kim's philosophy about life and her actions are grounded in this rebellious stance.

Similarly, Edouine described how she had defined herself against her mother. In this case, since her mother was not present, Edouine described how she had used her mother as a model of what not to be like. She said, "I know a lot of people feel like I'm not like my mother and I'm glad. I don't want to be like her." Edouine elaborated, "I don't want to be an alcoholic, have my man beating up on me, and people taking advantage of me, people spending my money, and me getting kicked out from place to place because of something silly."

Edouine's development involved comparing herself to her mother in order to be different. She said that her grandmother had compared Edouine to her mother and told her, "But you don't do what she does. You want to be smarter and intelligent and have a good job and she's going to sit home looking like a bum and an alcoholic." Edouine said she agreed that this was true and this motivated her to go to school.

Edouine described how she tested these issues with her mother. She said that she would point out that her mother hadn't gone to school and didn't have a job. Edouine stated her assessment of the situation: "I'd say, 'But she didn't do it. And she's my mother.' How can she tell me something if she didn't do it herself?" Edouine's comments indicate the importance of comparing her mother and herself. They also reveal her desire for her mother to be a positive role model.

Chantel defined herself as different from her mother in certain areas of her life. She seemed to question her likeness to her mother in terms of her own sanity; she had wondered whether she might ever be mentally ill. She said, "There were times in my life when I felt I was really going to go crazy. Sometimes I'd think I was on the edge of going really nuts." When asked how she had dealt with these fears, Chantel answered, "I'd think about the fact that I'm in college, that I have lots of things behind me."

Chantel said she also defined herself as different from her mother in her decision not to have an abortion. She said, "When I thought about abortion, I started thinking about how my parents were. I thought, 'If I have an abortion, I'd be rejecting this baby. That's just like my parents.'"

Her desire to be different from her mother was also part of her plans for her child's future. Chantel described talking to Stephen about his suggestion that the baby might be raised abroad by his family. She said:

> I told him, "You don't send a child away. You send mail away.
> "You send a package away, you know, you send letters away.

> "You don't send a child away." I said, "Your momma sent you away to your aunt and your grandmother. And my parents sent me away to go live in foster care." . . . I told him, "Hell no!" He better not ever mention that again.

Alicia said that in most areas of her life she was guided by her mother telling her what to do. However, in one area, her relationships with men, she said that she wanted to be different from her mother. Alicia said, "I used to say I wanted to be like my mom, be a nurse, but then what my stepfather put her through, people say, well, I'm going to grow up to have a husband beating up on me. Because I had that kind of environment around me. Personally, I don't think so. I know so."

However, as she continued, Alicia expressed strong doubts about whether it would be possible to achieve something different than her mother. She then said that she might have to avoid marriage; she continued, "I don't want nobody hitting on me. I just don't want to have no marriage like that. I said I was never ever going to get married so I don't have to worry about that."

This theme did not hold for Tanya or Shamika. Tanya's discussions did not feature any definition of herself as different from her mother. However, she did compare herself to her mother and questioned how they were similar. In discussing her pregnancy, Tanya noted that she and her mother—and grandmother and great-grandmother—were similar in having children young. She questioned the possible connection between this and her own pregnancy. I speculate that issues of comparison and differentiation might have emerged as a theme for Tanya had we had more interviews.

Shamika presented herself as being similar to her mother in many areas. She described her relationship with her mother as mostly positive; in particular, she said that she and her mother agreed on most things. She said that her mother deferred to Shamika's judgment in most instances. It seemed that Shamika was invested in seeing herself, and/or portraying herself, as very much united with her mother. Shamika's comments seemed to reflect a lack of separation or individuation from her mother.

Reflections on the Themes About Mothers

The participants described their mothers as having exerted significant influence on their lives; in particular, the effects of their mothers' absences or failings had been felt acutely. However, the equanimity with which the participants described the circumstances of their abandonment, rejection, and at times cruelty was striking. In part, this seemed due to a sense of acceptance or forgiveness of their mothers, perhaps out of an awareness of the mothers' difficult circumstances. This finding appears consistent with Elise's (1995) study, which found that black adolescent mothers, in comparison with white and Native American adolescent mothers, were more likely to identify with their mothers' struggles for survival than to blame them for their circumstances. However, this finding is contradicted by other research.[1]

It seemed these participants' experiences of the stresses of life may have given them the insight, or wisdom, to accept their mothers' failings. Gwaltney (1980) presented an ethic among black Americans that there is no sense in complaining or wishing things were otherwise because they're not. The participants' comments about their mothers suggest an accepting posture. However, they also raised questions about their mothers. It seemed they struggled to understand their mothers' feelings and actions, particularly those that had resulted in harm.

In spite of their experiences of having been rejected or failed by their mothers, most seemed to want some connection with them. They attempted to do this while protecting themselves from unrealistic expectations.

The finding that these young women's mothers were important in their lives and their discussions of their pregnancies is consistent with much of the literature on women's development[2] and an emerging body of literature on black mother-daughter relationships.[3] According to these theories, mothers are seen as forces from whom daughters struggle to separate and at the same time maintain connection with. From these perspectives, childbearing may be seen as a further issue of connection to, and separation from, one's mother.

This is seen most clearly in the cases of two participants—Alicia and Kim—who said that their mothers were directly involved in their decisions about pregnancy. Alicia complied with, and Kim rebelled against, the mother's wishes. Their resolutions support literature that suggests that adolescent pregnancy involves issues of autonomy and affiliation within the mother-daughter relationship (Jacobs, 1994).

However, the other four participants, whose mothers were not directly involved, also described their pregnancies in relation to their mothers. This suggests that the connection between the participants' mothers and their pregnancies is greater than the dynamics of the individual mother-daughter relationship.

Two of the participants with absent mothers—Edouine and Tanya—said that their mothers had, as adolescents, had children. This is consistent with literature that suggests an association between adolescent childbearing and one's mother's age at first birth.[4]

Some researchers (Gibbs, 1992) have suggested that transgenerational patterns of early childbearing may involve some form of role modeling. Even though a mother might not want her daughter to "repeat her mistake" of early childbearing (Ladner & Gourdine, 1984), the futility of "Do as I say, but not as I did" is apparent. This truth was discussed by Tanya. However, Tanya's observation seemed to have little impact on her plans for her own children. She said, "That cycle of having babies young has to stop. I don't want my child to be pregnant as a teenager. I don't. I really want to stress that. If I have to lock her up or lock him up, I'm going to. I don't want them getting pregnant young."

Although the dynamics of how patterns of early childbearing may be passed transgenerationally remain unclear, it seems important to acknowledge that these mother-daughter relationships were also influenced by the stresses the mothers experienced. These stresses included alcoholism, domestic violence, drug addiction, mental illness, and poverty.

Comparisons between the participants and their mothers were common throughout the participants' discussions. It might be that their pregnancies stirred thoughts about themselves in relation to their own mothers. Such reflections have been identified as part of many women's experiences of pregnancy.[5] These comparisons may also be understood in the context of literature that addresses the dynamics of mother-daughter relationships. Writing about white adolescent girls, Herman and Lewis (1984) suggested that, in adolescence, anger at one's mother reaches a peak. At that time, "young women express the greatest scorn for their mothers, the greatest desire to be different from their mothers, and the greatest fear that they will turn out to be just like their mothers" (p. 156). The participants' views of their mothers as expressed in the two themes seem to support this assessment. However, further exploration of the dynamics of black mother-daughter relationships is needed. Preliminary research by Cauce et al. (1996) on African American mothers and their adolescent daughters suggests that these relationships are characterized by struggle, conflict, and closeness, whereas Kaplan's (1997) ethnographic work with adolescent mothers suggests their relationships were marked by tension and alienation.

Pregnancy and adolescence may have contributed to participants' increased reflection on the similarities and differences between themselves and their mothers. However, it seemed that comparisons between themselves and their mothers had helped these young women define their goals and their identities throughout their lives.

Most participants said that they had used their mothers as negative examples of "what not to do" in at least one aspect of their lives. Edouine's comments exemplify this. Edouine said, "I know a lot of people feel like I'm not like my mother and I'm glad. I don't want to be like her." Most of the participants said that they had been successful in achieving more than their mothers, or in being different from them. The participants' successes seemed remarkable given the obstacles their mothers had experienced, which the participants had avoided. These include dropping out of school, alcoholism, substance abuse, mental illness, and physical abuse.

In general, the significance of mothers as role models cannot be overemphasized. As Edouine said about her mother, "How can she tell me something if she didn't do it herself?" Greene (1990) identified the pivotal influence of mothers as role models in African-American children's socialization. The importance of role models and identification with one's same-sex parent have been asserted as primary influences in identity definition at adolescence for black adolescent girls (Smith, 1982). It is noteworthy that only one participant mentioned other role models. It seemed there were few alternative role models available to the participants.

Although mothers as negative models may suffice to a certain point, in the absence of other influences, the effectiveness of this construct may run out. It seems it may be too difficult to succeed beyond a certain point—the point at which they got pregnant—perhaps because the next step is unimaginable. Collins (1990) identified that black girls are often helped to "go farther than [their] mothers themselves were allowed to go" (p. 54). However, without their mothers' and others' support, they may only be able to go so far. Given the fact that they have defined themselves by "not doing" what their mothers did, it may be too difficult to continue envisioning themselves differently, "successfully" in middle-class terms, in the absence of significant support. In a similar vein, Musick (1993) has suggested that ambivalence about separating more fully from their mothers and significant others may prompt pregnancy among lower-income girls. Kaplan's work (1997) also discusses these issues, suggesting the importance of class differences in the girls' socialization experiences and their relationships with their mothers.

For several of the participants, reflections on their mothers informed their hopes for the future. Kim, Edouine, Chantel, and Tanya noted an awareness of their mothers' limitations and said that they believed that they would do a better job in raising their own children. For Chantel this meant "I won't send my child away like I was," and for Kim, "I'll tell them the truth about things." These participants hoped to make up or correct the mothering they were given through raising their own children. This seems like a hopeful move, though how successful they will be is questionable.

Notes

1. Kaplan's (1997) study with black adolescent mothers indicated their expectation to be mothered in spite of an awareness of their mothers' circumstances.
2. Gilligan (1982) and Chodorow (1978).
3. Bell-Scott and Guy-Sheftall (1991) and Jacobs (1994).
4. Hogan and Kitagawa (1985), for example.
5. Chodorow (1978) and Gilligan (1982).

5

Balancing Hope and Pragmatism

Relationships with the Babies' Fathers

I Want the Baby's Father's Support/I Could Do Without It

This theme was true for three of the six participants. Kim, Shamika, and Edouine expressed this perspective on their partners' support. On the one hand, they said that they wanted their partners' involvement. They said they had hoped and expected that their partner would be supportive if they got pregnant. Once pregnant, they continued to want his involvement and would accept whatever support, emotional and/or financial, he is willing to provide. On the other hand, these participants said that, faced with the possibility of not having the partner's support, they could do without it.

The tension between these two sentiments—"I want his support" and "I could do without it"—seemed to suggest a balancing of their hope and desire for support with some pragmatism about having to manage without it. For these three participants, it seemed their saying they didn't need his support might be a way of preparing for, and/or protecting themselves against, this possibility.

These three expressed their wishes for their partner's support and simultaneously minimized its importance to them. Although Kim stated an unequivocal desire for Colin's support, she downplayed this in light of his noninvolvement. She said, "I would like him to be there, but I can't rely on that." She said that she maintained hope that Colin would change, while telling herself that she shouldn't count on this. Although she negated the likelihood of his support, Kim's comments revealed a fantasy she had about their future: "I can't say that he will marry me and pay for my college education and everything. You can't do that. . . . You can't plan what another person is going to do. . . . If it happens, then it will make my life easier."

She elaborated, "I still can't help but daydream. I daydream that one day Colin will fall in love with me again and take care of me and the baby and forget about all the other girls." About this recurrent fantasy, Kim said, "I guess it's to make me feel better. . . . Maybe to make me feel less abandoned. Like maybe one day he will get his act together. . . . It's just daydreaming, though, we'll see what happens."

Shamika simultaneously presented two opposing views about the importance of the father of the baby. She said that she had terminated a prior pregnancy because that partner had not been supportive. Her assessment that Jamal would be a good father was important in her decisions about this pregnancy. However, at the same time, she said that Jamal was not that important—that she was responsible for the decision to maintain the pregnancy. She said that she would be prepared if he decided not to be involved.

Her discussion featured mixed messages about Jamal's importance. Shamika said, "Jamal's been there all the other times so I think I can take a chance with him." About the pregnancy, Shamika assessed, "The decision about the pregnancy is really up to me. But it's both of our responsibility, so I think he should have a say-so. But if I didn't like his say-so, then I wouldn't do it! If he told me to have an abortion, I wouldn't go through it." She concluded, "So, in a way, he's important, but in a way, he's not. If he decided he didn't want to be bothered, I'd be prepared for it." She said this was important "because when you're having a baby you've gotta learn that the father might not always be there."

She related this attitude to a family teaching. Shamika explained, "That's a saying from my great-grandmother: 'A man can't do more for you than what you can do for yourself.' They preach that you can do much more than a man can do, rather than sitting around waiting for a man to do it for you." This teaching was based in a reality that "men can't really do nothing for you unless they got a job."

Edouine expressed a desire for Khary's involvement. She struggled with wanting to count on his support while having doubts about it. Edouine's evaluation that Khary was a good father had contributed to her wanting to have a baby with him. She said, "Khary was like 'How would you feel if I got you pregnant?' I said, 'I guess it would be no problem as long as I know you'd be there to take care of the child, that'd be no problem.'"

However, during the pregnancy, she began to doubt his ability to support her and their child. She was especially concerned about Khary's involvement with his three other children and their mothers. When confronted by his lack of support, Edouine said that she didn't need it. Edouine summarized her new perspective: "It takes two to have it, but it only takes one to raise it. Me. Because mostly it's just the mother raising it. The father, he's there, but he don't do everything the mother do."

The other three participants, Tanya, Chantel, and Alicia, did not contribute to this theme. Tanya and Chantel stated both a desire and a need for their partners' support. Unlike the three previously presented participants, they did not seem to be facing or contemplating the possibility that their partners might not be involved.

Although Tanya and Chantel said they had faced this possibility upon learning they were pregnant, they had no reason to believe their partners' support would not be forthcoming. They were currently dependent on their partners and said that their partners' support was essential. Perhaps the fact that they were receiving their partners' support freed them from a need to qualify their assessment of its importance.

Tanya said that she had confronted the possibility of not having Kahleem's support when she told him she was pregnant. She described that she had decided that, with or without his involvement, she would keep the pregnancy. However, she said she was very relieved to have his support. Tanya said, "I feel a little better, a little more secure than I was. . . . Because without him, I don't know what I'd be doing right now, who knows. Because he did a lot for me, stood by my side."

Chantel said she had been devastated by Stephen's nonsupportive response to learning that she was pregnant. When she told him, he had told her, "Do whatever you want to do," which she interpreted as meaning that she should have an abortion. She described her reaction: "At that moment, when I felt like I didn't have his support, I felt like 'I don't believe this.' I was flabbergasted. 'Now what?'" She said that she had been counting on his support; she was very relieved when his response changed. She elaborated, "I felt like 'Thank God, I have his support.'" Chantel's plans for the future included Stephen; she said that she was counting on having his support.

Alicia's situation differed from that of the other participants. During her pregnancy, Alicia had neither contact nor support from Alex, the father of the baby. Nearing the end of her pregnancy, after she told Alex she would keep the baby, he told her that he wanted to be involved. Unlike the other participants, Alicia said that she neither desired nor needed his involvement. The difference between Alicia and the other participants may be due to the fact that she had adjusted to his noninvolvement early on and had had little expectation that he would be a part of the pregnancy or the future.

However, after contact with Alex, near the end of her pregnancy, Alicia said she had decided she would allow his involvement. She said she did this primarily out of obligation. However, she restated her position that she didn't need his support. Alicia said, "He says he'll send money but I don't need his money, he don't have to. If he wants to, he can, but if he don't, it don't matter. That's the way I feel—if he wants to be there, he can, but if he don't, he don't."

Something About Him Just Attracted Me

This was a theme for Tanya, Kim, and Edouine. They said that there was something they couldn't explain that had attracted them to their partners. They described having had an initial physical attraction and then developing an emotional connection.

Tanya described her initial attraction to Kahleem. She said, "He's not the type of guy I would go for. It's something about him that attracted me to him when I first saw him. His smile was the first thing. He has the most prettiest smile. I tell him that all the time: 'You have the prettiest smile. That's a sexy smile.'"

Her descriptions of Kahleem featured his physical appearance and the fact that he was different from the types of men she had been involved with previously. Tanya said she couldn't explain why their relationship had evolved.

Kim similarly said there was something she couldn't explain involved in her attraction to Colin. She said, "Colin definitely made an impression on me right away. I don't believe in love at first sight, but it was just something about him." Her account of Colin also featured a physical description: "He's basically light-skinned. He was tall, nice build, and everything. He had his hair in extensions back then." She described how they met and how their relationship developed. She explained, "We became close on a mental level and we would talk about a lot of things."

Edouine's descriptions of her attraction to Khary featured an emotional connection. When asked what attracted her to Khary, Edouine said, "He made me laugh. Every time I was down and sad or had a problem I could always talk to him. He was like my brother more than my boyfriend. We was more buddies than boyfriend and girlfriend."

He's a Knucklehead

This statement, although uniquely voiced by Kim, expressed a sentiment that was true for Chantel, Shamika, and Edouine. These four participants presented pragmatic assessments of the babies' fathers' shortcomings. Although these participants openly expressed their dissatisfaction, it was mixed with resignation. They stated an acceptance of the partners' lifestyle; it seemed that there were things which they felt powerless to change that they must deal with.

Kim's reaction to Colin's lack of involvement in the pregnancy included resignation that her hopes were not being met. In describing Colin, she listed several things that were problems in their relationship with a certain acceptance. Kim described, "He's turning twenty-three this month and he doesn't really have a home, he sleeps at girlfriends' houses and everything. . . . He has another child; he didn't know about the other child 'til she was born."

Chantel's description of her relationship with Stephen included physical violence. Her explanation of this element was matter-of-fact. She said, "I have to say we fight a lot, and we get into physical fights." She stated, "This is bad for the baby, the unborn baby. . . . I want to trust him [Stephen] but . . . I don't."

Edouine's descriptions of Khary contained conflicting assessments. Edouine said, "He's nice. He's not like violent, sometimes he lets things go by, ease on by, but other times, if you press him the wrong way, he's not nice about it. But on the other hand, he's real nice. He's nice." Edouine elaborated that he sometimes became violent, but that he didn't mean to. She excused his behavior with her assessment that "he doesn't know what he's doing." She expressed concern about Khary, simultaneously negating her own perceptions.

Although she was aware of his flaws, she seemed to accept these as a part of their relationship. Edouine reported, "A lot of people think he's irresponsible. Sure, he is irresponsible if he got three kids by three different women, and then he going to have a fourth child by a fourth woman, and he lives with one of his babies' mother." She also noted, "He's in jail. I don't know when he going to come out, and I don't think he going to be out before the baby is born."

Shamika's description of her relationship with Jamal included her accepting reaction to his possessiveness. She said, "Sometimes he can be a pain, but that's part of dealing with it. He doesn't let me go anywhere because he feels that somebody else is going to want me. I don't mind because I want to be with him."

This theme did not hold for Alicia or Tanya. Alicia expressed dissatisfaction with Alex's response to her decision to put the baby up for adoption. However, she neither sought nor had contact with him during the pregnancy, and he was not involved. However, in her last interview, she said she would accept his involvement despite her reservations. Tanya did not express views on this issue in our interview.

He Don't Want No Stupid Baby Mother

Two participants, Shamika and Edouine, said that their partners stressed that the young women should continue their education. In both cases, it seemed unclear whether their partners were concerned about how a lack of education would reflect on the fathers or on their children.

Shamika said about Jamal, "He don't want no stupid baby mother." She expressed no reaction to Jamal's demand. However, Edouine said that she liked Khary's concern. Both participants said that when they got involved with their partners they had not been going to school and were unmotivated to continue school. Edouine said that Khary had told her, "I don't want no high school dropout." She elaborated, "He wants me to finish high school before the baby is born. He was like 'While you pregnant, go to school, go get your GED or something. . . . You finish school and go to college or you go to school and take up a trade or something.'" She described her reaction to his statements: "He's very strict on school. That's one thing I like about him because he won't let me go downhill."

Our Relationship's Not the Way I Thought It Would Be

Two of the participants, Kim and Edouine, spoke of how their relationships with their partners had changed during their pregnancies. They expressed feelings of disillusionment because they were not getting the support they had sought and expected. In light of this, Kim and Edouine questioned their prior assessments about the pregnancy, their relationship, their partner, and themselves. As a result, they expressed feelings of resignation and self-blame. Their accounts suggest the differences in expectations and assessments between themselves and their partners. These also indicate differences between their own expectations and assessments before and after the pregnancy.

Kim's realization that her relationship with Colin was not what she had hoped made her question the basis of their relationship and her judgment. She assessed, "I did feel like he cared about me back in those days. It's not the same anymore. Back then I did feel he cared about me. I think he probably did."

Kim said that she blamed herself:

> For allowing myself to go through this situation as long as I did. Then again, I guess I was in love, too. So, I kind of blame myself for my staying and being with him. I was kind of stupid for letting my emotions get away with myself. I guess people thought I was stupid, too. I guess I am in terms of staying with and still sleeping with him and listening to him when he said he loved me. Now I don't believe that.

Her evaluation included a negative assessment of herself: "If I was smart enough I wouldn't have gotten so involved with him and been pregnant now."

Although Kim stated an awareness of differences between her previous expectations and the current reality, she still maintained some hope that things might change. She said:

> I still love Colin. You can't help loving your baby's father because you had a relationship. You have a piece of him inside you kicking you every few hours. You can't help still feeling emotions for the baby's father. I'm trying to put that on the back burner. I have a feeling that you can't change somebody. They have to change themselves basically.

Edouine's account of her relationship with Khary changed near the end of her pregnancy when they broke up. She described: "I don't know what happened. He just stopped calling me. Me and him just didn't agree on a lot of things about the baby. And I felt I was getting everything for the baby and he wasn't trying to do nothing so I felt, I don't need that. If that was the case, I can do it all by myself."

This development influenced her assessment of their relationship and the pregnancy. Although she had previously said that she and Khary had discussed pregnancy and agreed it was something they wanted, she now presented a different aspect. Edouine explained, "Khary wanted to get me pregnant. I didn't want to get pregnant because I knew that I didn't have a steady place where I was living." She said her feelings changed: "Gradually the thought of it, having my own baby and all, it seemed it would be nice."

Edouine described how this also changed once she was pregnant. She said that she suddenly thought about not having a place to live and not having finished her education. She elaborated, "That was really something that I was really worried about when I got pregnant, but it wasn't really nothing when we was doing it without a condom." In hindsight, she presented an assessment of how this happened:

> I must have been thinking about making him happy instead of doing what I had to do for myself. I didn't want to make him feel like, no, I didn't want to have a baby. I didn't know what to do 'cause if I didn't give it to him, somebody else would. That's how I was feeling. I felt like he was going to find somebody else if he don't get me pregnant or we don't do what we have to do or something like that. I think that's all why I just let him stop using a condom or whatever.

In retrospect she questioned his motives and actions, and her judgment. Edouine elaborated, "I felt like he must have been joking at the time. I never thought that he would lie to me. Now I feel like everything he was telling me was lies—about marriage, and that he want to be with me and live with me."

The resulting assessment of her situation was negative: "I feel like I got used, like he got what he wanted. He got me pregnant and got what he wanted out of me and just left. I felt real bad." Edouine said she was depressed: "I got disgusted and I just stay in my room by myself."

Reflections on the Themes About the Babies' Fathers

The participants made contradictory statements about the importance of the fathers of their babies. This is illustrated by the primary theme: "I want his support/I could do without it." On the one hand, most described having had an investment in the prepregnancy relationship with these partners and wanting to maintain this relationship. This investment contradicts popular notions that these were casual liaisons and that the young women were, as Alicia commented, "just out to get pregnant." The participants' descriptions of their early relationships are contained in the theme "Something about him just attracted me." All of the participants described an emotional involvement with a partner whom they cared about and with whom they had considered pregnancy. Their summaries contain elements similar to those described in the literature about love (e.g., Sternberg, 1986).

Several of the participants said that although they had previously used birth control or had ruled out the possibility of maintaining a pregnancy, something about this relationship was different. They said they could not identify or describe this difference; Kim's comments about her relationship with Colin are illustrative. She said, "I started to think that I could have his baby. . . . Somehow it was different with Colin. . . . I had very strong feelings for him."

In discussing their early relationships, the participants said that their partners had offered something they didn't have. For most, this was friendship, humor, and support; these seemed especially important given the participants' histories and their circumstances at that time. Although the participants' statements and situations varied, Chantel was particularly straightforward about her circumstances. She said, "When Stephen, my boyfriend, came along, I wanted to take advantage of the situation. I was thinking, 'He really loves me, let me kinda like hop on this. This could be my ticket out of the group home.' In a way, I was using him, but I thought it could be good."

In most cases, their partners provided attention, support, and an opportunity or hope for a better life. The participants described their fantasies about what they wanted and what they had thought their relationships with the fathers would be like. They shared their dreams about their relationship and the future. This is consistent with Anderson's (1993) findings. Anderson described, "The dream involves having a boyfriend, a fiance, a husband, and the fairy-tale prospect of living happily ever after in a nice house in a neighborhood with one's children—essentially the dream of the middle-class American life-style" (p. 79).

Anderson (1993) suggested these fantasies are instrumental in influencing relationships among lower-income black adolescents and often precipitate out-of-wedlock adolescent pregnancy. My findings suggest some support for Anderson's views; however, the situation is more complex for the young women involved than he implied. All of the participants said that they had talked about the possibility of pregnancy with their partner. Kim, Edouine, Chantel, and Tanya said that they had discussed this in terms of a "what if" scenario. They had talked with their partners saying, "What if I got pregnant?" As Tanya said:

> Kahleem and I had talked about getting pregnant before. . . . We talked about how we wanted to have a baby after we bought a house, after we got everything established, so we'd have something to fall back on. We had thought about what if it happened now. But we was like, we ain't going to let that happen.

The participants said they felt that their partners had known about, and had agreed to take, the risk of pregnancy. They said they had believed that if they got pregnant their partners would be supportive. However, they said that they had also considered the possibility that they might not be able to count on this support and had decided to maintain the pregnancy anyhow.

It seems important that all of the participants mentioned their familiarity with single parenting through their family and friends. Their contextual experiences of single mothers and of female households seemed to exert influence on their views of marriage and childbearing (Gibbs, 1992). These realities are part of what is learned when growing up. As Gibbs (1992) suggested, girls raised in homes where a mother is a self-sufficient household head may receive the implicit message that husbands are not essential to establish and raise a family. This may be further reinforced by attitudes, values, and behaviors of peers and siblings (Gibbs, 1992).

Although the participants may dream of something different, they were taught to be prepared for an alternative reality. This is evidenced by Shamika's description of a family teaching. She described that the lesson—"A man may not be able to do more for you than you can do for yourself"—had been handed down through generations. This is consistent with Collins's (1991) and others'[1] findings about black mothers teaching their daughters the importance of self-reliance and resourcefulness.

Many researchers, including Franklin (1992), Ladner (1971), and W. J. Wilson (1987), have addressed the high rates of single parenthood, female-headed households, and birth outside of marriage in lower-SES black communities. Multiple reasons have been suggested for how and why these family patterns evolved. W. J. Wilson (1987), for example, identifies economic changes resulting in a lack of jobs that deprive young men of the opportunity to prove their manhood by supporting a family and foster a dependence on public assistance by single mothers. However, others[2] reject this assessment, citing more complex historical, structural, and psychological influences.

In spite of an awareness of the poor prospects for male employment, and their families' teachings, the participants seemed willing to take a chance in their relationships with the babies' fathers. This is perhaps because of what their partner offered them (e.g., attention, love) and, in part, because of what they hoped their relationship would bring in the future.

The tension between their fantasies and the possible opposite reality may explain the contradiction of their statements about their partners' importance. While stating their wish, "I'd like his support," they are at the same time trying to protect themselves from disappointment—"I could do without it." Such a self-protective strategy seems appropriate within this context. Although the participants who have their partners' support can talk freely about how much it means to them and how they need it, those who may not are more guarded.

The participants' desire to believe in this fantasy and to hold onto or achieve this relationship is suggested by their willingness to accept their partners in spite of their dissatisfactions. This is reflected in the theme "He's a knucklehead." In addition, the importance of meeting their partners' demands is suggested by "He don't want no stupid baby mother." These themes may also reflect a relationship of antagonism and love between partners. Collins (1990) discussed this as the "love and trouble tradition" of relations between black women and men.

Even when the participants may see discrepancies between their fantasies and reality, they may refuse to accept evidence of a less optimistic situation. They are clearly invested in maintaining their beliefs. This seems understandable considering their situation of being pregnant by this partner.

The views of two participants, Edouine and Kim, who confronted disappointing realities are expressed in the theme "Our relationship is not the way I thought it would be." Their comments indicated how their feelings and assessments changed over time as they struggled to accommodate the reality that the partner was not involved the way they had thought he would be. This development led to a reassessment of their relationship, the partner's motives, and their own judgment and participation. In the end, it seemed self-blame resulted; as Kim said, "I guess I was foolish for letting myself get carried away."

Several participants mentioned that marriage to the baby's father was neither necessary nor sought. This seems consistent with a general norm of not getting married to the fathers of their babies.[3] This finding may be interpreted in light of the scarcity of men available for marriage in this context[4] as well as cultural norms.[5]

However, most of the participants were receiving some support from their partners. The participants said that, although they did not believe in marriage, they were glad to have their partners' support. As Tanya said, "Right now, the only one I have is Kahleem. . . . Without him, I don't know what I'd do." All of the participants planned to maintain some relationship with the father of the baby. These intentions, whether or not they are realized, are consistent with research suggesting that there may be strong, if not legal, ties between parents in lower-SES black communities.[6]

Notes

1. Carothers (1990).
2. See Brewer (1995) and Kaplan (1997), among others.
3. See Adams, Pittman, and O'Brien (1993); Franklin (1992); and Rhoden and Robinson (1997).
4. W. J. Wilson (1987).
5. Dickerson (1995) and P. M. Wilson, (1986).
6. Furstenberg, Brooks-Gunn, and Morgan (1987) and Way and Stauber (1996).

6

Confronting Difference

Their Experiences of "Race"

Because I'm Darker, Is My Heart Different?

This theme reflects the participants' discussions about race that emerged for four of the six participants. Tanya, Chantel, Alicia, and Kim talked about race issues; in particular, they spoke of their experiences of racial discrimination.

These participants' comments revealed an acute awareness of people's reactions to their appearance in terms of race. It seemed they struggled to develop and maintain a sense of unique identity and self-esteem in spite of their experiences of discrimination and racism. They seemed optimistic about equality and believed that they would have opportunities for achievement. These hopeful comments, in spite of their experiences to the contrary, seemed poignant. Their discussions also contained questions about why racism and discrimination exist.

The following four participants discussed issues related to their racial/ethnic identity. Tanya described that she had experienced people's reactions to her light-colored skin. Tanya said that her mother had very dark skin and her father was white. She explained that she was "the lightest thing" in her family. She said that people often doubted that she was her mother's daughter due to the difference in their skin colors. She reported that when people reacted to this, she responded that it was none of their business. She said, "A human being is only a human being, 'cause you take everybody's skin off, we all have red blood. Word up [truth]. I don't even worry about it."

Tanya said that both black and white people had reacted negatively to her skin color. She said, "The blacks treated me like I was an outcast because they called me traitor. 'How could you turn the white way?' I say,

'Well, I was born this way, how can I do anything about it?' The white man is like 'Well, you want to be honky.' . . . I was like, I don't care about anybody. I'm a human being."

She described a racial incident at school in which students fought. When a student had asked which side she belonged on, Tanya replied, "I'm on my own side. I don't care what you all do, kill each other, whatever, but I'm the one who will be still living and getting my education."

Chantel discussed her experience of racial discrimination when she was refused a job. She said, "I just left. I didn't even want to bother with it. Because I feel that it's just going to make everything worse." She described the effect of this experience of racism. She said, "It doesn't discourage me, it only encourages me. I just say, the hell with you, you missed out on me. That's how I feel now. Because I've been rejected a lot, so now it's like 'Well, you missed out. I'm a damn good cashier or whatever. You missed out, not me.'"

Chantel also presented thoughts about the issue of discrimination, saying:

> I'm not an animal. Why treat me differently because I'm just darker. What's the big deal? Okay, I'm darker. Because I'm darker is my heart different from yours? Does my heart pump differently from yours? Are my eyes different? I mean, do your eyes contain something my eyes don't? I don't think anybody is better than me. That's how I am, and I don't think I'm better than anybody else. I hate when people, you know, try to discriminate because of color. I think that it's so stupid.

Chantel's thoughts included larger questions about how racial discrimination and prejudice evolved. She speculated that "something must have happened a very long time ago." She noted that racist ideas about superiority could just as easily have evolved to be biased in favor of dark-colored skin.

Alicia's discussion of issues related to race focused on negative perceptions about black females who got pregnant. She said, "I used to look down on girls who used to do that, especially the black females. That's what everybody's expecting from them, to have babies and stuff." She elaborated the influence of this stereotype on her self-perceptions, saying that now that she was pregnant she was "another statistic." Alicia said that she did not want to see herself that way.

She described how her attitudes about race were influenced by her mother and her upbringing. She said that there had been only four black children in her elementary school. She said, "I was the only black kid achieving in school, so the black kids tried to put me down. They thought

I wanted to be with the white people. Because I am trying to make the same standards as the white kids." She said that she concentrated on her work and didn't take it personally.

Alicia discussed discrimination and said she disagreed with her friend's belief that a white person would get a job faster than a black person. She said, "If you have the education and the right status, I think the black person could get it as well as the white person." Alicia presented her philosophy: "If you think you're doing the right thing, just go on and do it."

Kim's experiences about race dealt with others' reactions to her. She explained, "Because I'm part Chinese and black, people would look at me differently and stuff because I didn't exactly look like one or the other." She described an incident from her childhood when two black women had exclaimed outrage about "a young child [Kim] traveling by herself on the train" although she was seated next to her mother.

Kim also recounted a more personal experience of her mother's reactions to her. She described:

> My mother didn't know how to raise a black American child. Like when it came to my hair, she'd just say, "Ugh, your hair." She didn't really know what to do with it. Once in a while, the girls in my neighborhood would go and braid my hair for me. But, other times, my mom would just end up cutting off all my hair so I had an Afro. She did that twice; that's why I don't let her touch me, ever again, when it comes to hair and other things.

Kim also described some white people's reactions to her. She said growing up she had hung around the "rich white people" whose houses her mother cleaned. She said this made her question how they felt about her and how she felt about herself. In addition, she spoke about her experiences of going to a private school on scholarship. She said, "Basically, since we're on scholarship, it's like you don't belong here anyway. That's why a lot of the black students left."

Reflection on the Theme About Race

I was surprised by the amount and depth of material that emerged about race. Because I was exploring pregnancy, I had not expected participants to discuss issues related to this topic. That they did caused me to wonder whether the participants' talking about their experiences of discrimination and views about race were related to my being white. This is a reasonable possibility. However, in part, the emergence of this topic may be due to the effective use of ethnographic interviewing, in which topics of relevance to the participants are addressed.

I believe the discussions of race might also have emerged because it is a relevant part of their life experience. The studies of Gwaltney (1980) and Ladner (1971) suggested that the experience of institutionalized racial oppression is a pervasive influence in black Americans' lives, one with which the participants seem to grapple. The participants' comments may also reflect the fact that, developmentally, they are struggling to define themselves as black Americans (Phinney & Rosenthal, 1992; Ward, 1990).

The participants' comments about race may be viewed within the context of racial identity literature.[1] Parham (1989), among others,[2] elaborated a model of Nigresence, or the psychological process of becoming black. Parham suggested that various stages of racial identity development occur over the life span. He argued that these stages reflect one's attempts to balance Afro-American and Euro-American values within one's life.

Viewed within Parham's (1989) model of racial identity development, the participants' comments seem to reflect predominantly "preencounter" attitudes. In this frame, the participants expressed attitudes characterized by "an idealistic/humanistic perspective in which Blackness is denied in favor of assimilation and being accepted as 'just a human being'" (p. 199). Tanya's and Chantel's comments fit with this pattern. Parham suggested that individuals in this stage deny social realities and view their lives as if racism were nonexistent.

However, the participants' comments suggested that they also contemplate their experiences and question larger social issues, including racism. In light of Parham's (1989) model, these comments may reflect the beginnings of movement between stages as the participants experienced significant events that were inconsistent with their frame of reference. However, this was not explored in our interviews and I am hesitant to speculate about their experience. In a future study, it would be interesting to explore whether or how participants believed their pregnancies influenced how they saw themselves and how they were seen. Alicia's contemplation of her pregnancy in relation to racial stereotypes suggested that by becoming pregnant, she moved into a particular stereotype associated with her race, age, and gender.[3]

All of these participants seemed to grapple with issues related to racial identity. It seemed they faced a difficult struggle to define who they are and where they fit. Several of the participants described experiences of discrimination by white, and black, people. Experiences of the latter were related to having light-colored skin and/or having parents from different ethnic/racial backgrounds.

This theme did not hold for Shamika or Edouine. This absence may reveal a belief that this issue was not relevant to our discussions, or it may reflect a lack of comfort in discussing issues related to race with me. It may also reflect the fact that race was not a significant issue for these participants at that time.

Notes

1. Cross (1991); Hall, Freedle, and Cross (1972); and Helms (1990), among others.
2. See Cross, Parham, and Helms (1991).
3. See Collins (1991) and Kaplan (1997).

7

Seeming Contradictions

The Complex Themes

The previous chapters present the themes that emerged from the analysis; these included three overarching paradoxical themes that were introduced in the groups of themes in Chapters 3 through 6. These paradoxical themes are (1) "It happened/I wanted it," (2) "I want the baby's father's support/I could do without it," and (3) "Once you're pregnant, you have to think about the future/I'm living day-to-day." To me, these themes seemed to be contradictions because they expressed beliefs that appear to oppose each other, although the participants did not present these as conflictual. In contemplating the meaning of these seeming contradictions, I was aware of engaging a perspective of "both/and" instead of "either/or," which, although not neat, would allow both parts of the seeming contradiction to be "true" at the same time.

In thinking about the meaning of these seeming contradictions, I considered what has been addressed as the "split subjectivities" of women (Fine & Zane, 1991). Researchers such as Fine and Zane (1991) and others (Collins, 1990; Harding, 1986; Riger, 1992) have suggested that women, due to their particular position in the social hierarchy, possess unique vantage points from which to view the world around them. In particular, low-income women of color may provide perspectives that are particularly meaningful due to these women's positioning "at the intersection of class, race, and gender oppression" (Fine & Zane, 1991, p. 86).

Such "split subjectivities" may also be related to the complexities inherent in being black and American. Du Bois (1903/1989) identified this as a "double consciousness" or "second sight." As Du Bois described, "One ever feels his twoness—an American, a Negro; two souls, two thoughts, two unreconciled strivings; two warring ideals" (p. 5).

Such "split subjectivities" may result in contradictory reflections such as those that Fine and Zane (1991) found in their discussions with minority girls of low income. Fine and Zane, relying on Harding (1986), identified that "what has historically been read as woman contradicting herself [may be reframed] as woman, from a position of disempowerment, viewing a world from both inside and from the margins"(p. 86).

These authors suggested that, through these contradictory reflections, the participants "merge their experience, their critiques and longings for what could be" (p. 88).

What appears to be contradictory in these complex themes may similarly be considered to reflect and embrace complexities of the young women's lives. Each of the contradictions may be reframed as an instance in which an espoused norm or belief—often society's "official version"—is at variance with the participants' own experiences. The latter must be considered in terms of the multiple layers of being black, female, and of lower income.

The participants' discussions support the fact that, on the one hand, they have been raised to believe that they must rely on themselves to get what they need. This is illustrated by the themes "I want the baby's father's support/I could do without it" and "Deal with it!" Their belief is consistent with research about self-reliance as part of the socialization of black females (Collins, 1990). In addition, the participants' experiences of life—including abandonment, chaos, and abuse—have shown them that they cannot rely on others.

On the other hand, the participants asserted that they had learned through experience that life is capricious and that they cannot assert much control over life events. This belief is conveyed by two aspects of the paradoxical themes: "It happened" as well as "I'm just living day-to-day." It seemed that, although they were asked to be agents in directing their lives, their experience informs them that their efforts are not effective. These two beliefs—that one must be self-reliant and that life is not within their control—seem both accurate and at odds. This dilemma reflects issues of women's agency raised by Riger (1992) and Stewart (1994). Riger (1992) noted the need to "link a vision of women's agency with an understanding of the shaping power of social context" (p. 738).

Similarly, the participants reflected on the fact that they were raised to believe that they should defer childbearing in order to achieve academic or career success. However, their comments revealed that these future goals seemed unreal (as Kim reflected, "It wasn't clear because it wasn't my path") and out of their control (as Edouine said about becoming a lawyer, "If it happens, it happens"). In addition, the views expressed were at variance with what they saw enacted around them: family and peers who, as adolescents, had had children. Additionally, it seemed the espoused ideal of deferring childbearing ignored the reality that through pregnancy the participants hoped to gain something they needed. To dismiss this is to deny their hard-learned knowledge that they must take advantage of every possible situation that comes their way that could get them what they need.

In addition, the participants' beliefs about their relationships with the babies' fathers are relevant. On the one hand, they need to take advantage of what comes their way, and they believe they will benefit from these relationships, yet, on the other hand, they have been taught they cannot rely on men. When the young women are disappointed in these relationships, it seems self-blame results; as Kim said, "I was kind of stupid for letting my emotions get away with myself."

The paradoxical theme "Once you're pregnant, you have to think about the future/I'm just living day-to-day" conveys the duality that although the participants needed to think about the future, they had to be prepared for something different to happen. In terms of making meaning of their pregnancies, they did so with a belief that their futures are uncertain. All of the participants mentioned that they had learned from past experience that because life is unpredictable, it would be foolish to count on something until it happens. As Alicia said, "I'm not thinking too far ahead. There's no use thinking too much and when the time comes, something else ends up happening." This is directly at variance with the belief that one should postpone childbearing in order to achieve another goal.

It seems noteworthy that none of the participants described pregnancy as interfering with her plans for the future; in fact, some participants suggested that pregnancy would help them reach their goals. This is consistent with recent research suggesting that the traditional assessment of negative educational outcomes due to adolescent pregnancy does not hold. Chantel's comments are illustrative. Chantel felt that pregnancy allowed her "time out" to decide what career she wished to pursue on returning to school. She said, "After I have the baby, I'll probably go to school two days a week and still be a full-time student. Or I might have to go to night school with the baby if Stephen can't help out."

This seems to suggest an attitude of optimism, or denial, which may be due to the fact that they were committed to maintaining their pregnancies. However, it may also reflect that within lower-SES black populations, the economic disadvantages associated with adolescent childbearing may be less severe than for those in other populations. Several recent studies have suggested that in this population early childbearers may not suffer the negative effects on education and income previously associated with adolescent childbearing (Geronimus & Korenman, 1990) or that they may make up these differences later in life (Furstenberg et al.,

1987). These researchers have suggested that within this population adolescent childbearing per se may not be the cause of negative economic and educational consequences.

The participants were optimistic that they would be able to survive with support from the baby's father, their family, and/or working or by unspecified means. However, most did not have any stable source of income or support. Their hopeful expectations about the future may reflect a belief that life is difficult but contains the possibility that things will get better. This sustaining belief has been identified as a pervasive influence in black Americans' cultural experience from slavery to the present (Gwaltney, 1980).

As a related issue, "I wanted it"—an element of the paradoxical theme about pregnancy—seems to suggest the participants' belief that there may be advantages to their pregnancies. However, contrary to popular belief, the participants' perceptions of any potential advantages did not include the anticipation of receiving welfare benefits. Rather, their perspectives seemed to suggest that any potential advantages were related to the dearth of attractive, realistic alternatives. This perspective is supported by researchers (Burden & Klerman, 1984; Williams & Kornblum, 1985) who have suggested that early childbearing is related to the lack of meaningful and equal career opportunities among lower-SES black teens. This is not to suggest that the consequences of adolescent childbearing are not difficult or are desirable. However, the impact of these consequences must be interpreted in light of their histories and the realities of their life circumstances.

The paradoxical themes as a group may be considered instances that reflect these young women's experiences of life and meaning making. Within this context, pregnancy may be seen as an attempt to resolve the ambiguities or contradictions they experience. Although these young women—because of their social class position, ethnicity, race, and gender—may have limited control over the larger forces that influence them, through their pregnancies, they may try to take some control. Rather than being powerless, they act to create what they believe will be better lives within circumstances of deprivation.

This perspective is based on an assumption that "within the context of relative powerlessness, women—like all people in a subordinate status—make choices and resist oppression" (Stewart, 1994, p. 23). Although it may sometimes be hard to recognize, some type of agency exists. As Fine (1989) assessed, "Persons of relatively low ascribed social power . . . cannot control those forces which limit their opportunities [but] they do assert control in ways ignored by psychologists" (p. 187).

In this frame, pregnancy may represent a viable way for these young women to get what they need. For some, pregnancy seems to be an attempt to burst through the contradictions they live—in particular, to deal with the conflict between the "espoused" norm versus the "real" norm, as well as knowledge based in their own experiences. It provides a means to confront, and resist, the realities that would render them confused and powerless. Although pregnancy is often seen as an act of relinquishing control, for some young women it may be an act of taking control.

This perspective does not dismiss the fact that these young women exhibited varying degrees of what might be considered "passivity" in their choices about childbearing. Some participants' choices seemed less "conscious" or "active." However, this view opens up the possibility that instances that may look like "giving up control" may, in fact, be "ways to survive" (Fine, 1989). As a related issue, Fine (1989) has argued that there is a need to "expand the definition of 'taking control' to incorporate the lived experience of women and men across class, race and ethnic lines" (p. 196).

In summary, this consideration of the paradoxical themes engages the complicated realities and beliefs that shape these young women's lives. The findings suggest that the meanings of pregnancy are socially constructed within a context of need and uncertainty. How they define themselves and the meanings of pregnancy are influenced by a combination of factors—their partners, their relationships with their mothers, an awareness of peers with babies, poor performance or lack of direction in school, and uncertainty about their plans for the future. That all of these play some role in the participants' having babies supports a contextual model of factors influencing childbearing. However, the issues involved are greater than just pregnancy and childbearing. It seemed these issues include the realities of inequality, poverty, and racism and their experiences of social structures that neither value nor address these young women's needs.

The perspective forwarded in this book suggests the importance of addressing multiple realities and meanings within a particular context. It is a unique way of conceptualizing these different influences. It includes the ambiguous, ambivalent, and conflictual aspects of becoming pregnant. In addition, it highlights the conditions of need and constraint that influence these young women. My perspective also engages the participants' philosophies about life, which underlie and influence their actions.

8

Implications for an Alternative Developmental Model

At the center of this book lie the stories of the six young women whose interviews revealed the inextricable link between their childbearing and their experiences of, and beliefs about, life. In the previous chapter, I addressed the complex themes to reflect the complicated realities and beliefs that shape these young women's lives. I considered what seemed to me to be contradictions—including how pregnancy just "happened" yet was something that they wanted—as a way to confront conflict between norms of mainstream culture and their own experiences and to get what they need. I argued that how they define themselves and the meanings of pregnancy are influenced by a combination of factors, including their partners, their relationships with their mothers, an awareness of peers with babies, poor performance or lack of direction in school, and uncertainty about their plans for the future. That all of these play some role in the participants' having babies supports a contextual model of factors influencing their childbearing. However, the issues involved are greater than just pregnancy and childbearing. These issues include the realities of inequality, poverty, racism, and discrimination, as well as social structures that neither value nor address these young women's needs. Through their pregnancies, all the participants, except Alicia, act to create what they believe will be better lives within limited circumstances.

In this chapter, I consider these young women's experiences as they suggest implications for an "alternative developmental model." The choice to do so is based on a belief in the "rationality" of their childbearing in light of how this fits together with their philosophies and realities of life. The term *alternative* is used primarily to mark the contrast with what is known about pathways of middle-class, predominantly white youth. However, it is also an "alternative" pathway that differs from that of the majority of urban adolescent girls of color who do not become adolescent mothers.

Implicit in my outlining of the implications of this perspective is a critique, or at least a question, about development as a linear progression toward some goal. Rather, the emphasis here is on exploring the conditions at this particular stage. This consideration rests on an acknowledgment that traditional assumptions of development as proceeding "toward" some preordained point may not apply (Walkerdine, 1993). In addition, it does not assume that "development" is predictive of any certain outcome (Lewis, 1997). Despite some criticism of definitions of "development" as "change,"[1] this definition must suffice for now insofar as it illuminates what is going on with these young woman, at this particular time in their lives. Certainly their pregnancies represent a time of intense "change" as they experience what has happened and anticipate what may happen following delivery.

Based on this study, a question arises as to what would be important to include in a developmental model that would help us to understand the experiences of these six young women participants. Building blocks for an alternative developmental model derived from the study of the participants' lives will be examined in the following section.

Engaging with the Voices and Experiences of Black Adolescent Girls to Learn About Their Development

Recent psychological research suggests that we have limited understanding of the developmental pathways of ethnic minority and economically disadvantaged teens. An emerging body of research suggests that the realities of life for adolescents within lower-SES urban black American communities contribute to developmental trajectories that differ from those of traditional, majority youth (Burton, Obeidallah, & Allison, 1996). Thus, there is a need for developmental models that start from, or at least incorporate, nonmajority experiences. It has been suggested that new paradigms may be necessary to guide this developmental research and that ethnographic accounts can provide key insights into these different developmental pathways (Jessor, Colby & Shweder, 1996).

The participants' data supported the need to consider a different developmental pathway that would apply to the participants and other adolescent girls in their context. As Tanya indicated, "Most of my friends have kids and some are already on their second child. . . . I was one of the last to become pregnant." The participants' interviews revealed complex perspectives on their pregnancies and their lives. In order to understand these perspectives it was necessary to learn more about their beliefs about life and the life experiences that informed these beliefs. The research process involved attending to multiple threads embedded in their narratives. These threads included the participants' personal histories, their expectations, and their beliefs about life. Here, the use of qualitative methods was invaluable. This study supports the need to learn of the possibilities of different developmental paths and processes by engaging with the voices of those involved.

The Differences in "*Adolescence*" in Different Contexts

Adolescence is commonly viewed as a time of preparation for adulthood, as a time "between" childhood and adulthood. However, as Ruddick (1993) notes, "The experience of 'adolescence,' although tied to bio-sexual maturity, varies by class, ethnicity, religious expectations, education and a host of other cultural factors" (p. 128). She notes that families and cultures of poor, black, and other nondominant groups may not recognize adolescence as a concept in the same way as the dominant culture.

Other researchers, including Ladner (1971), have identified that poor black children are not often granted the luxury of childhood or adolescence. It seems that although mainstream youth may experience adolescence as a time of increasing freedom of choice, adolescents in challenging circumstances tend to face increasing demands and limitations. Findings from this study suggest the need to consider the meaning of "adolescence" in light of the participants' life experiences. One needs to question whether or not these young women are afforded the luxury of adolescence. A strongly voiced theme was "Life is hard." Participants said this belief was informed by their experiences dealing with difficult family situations, challenging personal circumstances, and limited economic resources. Participants stated that they had had to grow up quickly and had been responsible for taking care of themselves for years. As Edouine said, "When I was thirteen, I just realized that I have to take care of myself because nobody else it going to do it for me."

Burton, Obeidallah, and Allison's (1996) summary of ethnographic works about adolescents in inner-city contexts noted a common finding is that of inconsistent role expectations: "For example, in school, these adolescents are often treated like 'older children' while at home they are treated like 'grown folks' saddled with adult responsibility" (p. 405). Thus, these adolescents experience contexts of development that differ greatly from those experienced by mainstream youth and those envisioned in traditional developmental models (e.g., Erikson's stages of identity). As Burton et al. (1996) suggest, "Mixed messages [about role expectations] may result in adolescence being considered an abridged or ambiguous developmental stage among teens who are struggling to survive in challenging environments" (p. 405).

Adolescent Tasks and Outcomes That May Differ from the Mainstream

Recent research on minority adolescents' development reflects an awareness of the need to incorporate new perspectives in assessing development among lower-income minority populations. Winfield (1995), for example, has argued the need to shift from the notion of "at risk" to that of "resilience" in studying African-American adolescents. There is also consensus that minority youths' development may include different tasks, for example, those related to ethnic identity (Phinney & Rosenthal, 1992). In addition to different tasks, some researchers have argued the need to incorporate different developmental outcomes for minority youth in poverty. It is unclear how, or even whether, developmental outcomes should be determined contextually.[2]

In approaching a model that acknowledges different tasks and outcomes among lower-income minority youth, direction may be taken from the model of child development forwarded by Almeida, Woods, and Messeneo (1998). Almeida et al.'s (1998) model highlights the intersecting influences of race, gender, class, and culture. In this model, the focus shifts from autonomy and traditional notions of achievement to a focus on children's development in different social roles. Almeida et al. define maturity as the "ability to live in respectful relation" (p. 23) to others and to a complex, multifaceted world. Their model includes developmental tasks related to interdependence such as respect for others and the ability to communicate and to collaborate.

A reconceptualization of tasks and outcomes would better suit the participants' data and would acknowledge capacities and achievements overlooked or ignored by traditional models. A reconceptualization might incorporate awareness of how participants survived and even thrived in spite of significant stressors. For example, some participants reported that staying in school and staying sane were important, difficult achievements. One participant, Chantel, talked about her struggles in light of her mother's mental illness and her father's abuse. She said, "There were times in my life when I felt I was really going to go crazy. Sometimes I'd think I was on the edge of going really nuts, because of a lot of things that happened to me. Especially when I was fighting with my father. But then I'd think about the fact that I'm in [school], that I have a lot of things behind me. I'd look at my grades—I have report cards with nineties and eighty-fives to show for what I did. That really backed me up."

Comments from another participant, Edouine, reveal another capacity—perhaps defined as connection or generosity—which may also represent an achievement. She questioned, "I wonder if I'm going to be the way I am now, always friendly and considerate to other people's needs and helping other people. Or will I just be looking out for myself."

The Need for a Culturally Variable, Expanded Definition of *Agency*

My analysis of the participants' interviews revealed the centrality and complexity of issues of agency. *Agency* has been defined as "a person's ability to experience wants and goals and to take action to pursue them" (Richardson, 1994, p. 40).[3] The data revealed the importance of agency not only in terms of pregnancy but in relation to other issues including the participants' plans for work/career and relationships. Engaging with agency is essential to considerations of development.

The findings about whether or how pregnancy was desired and/or sought were complicated. This complexity is expressed in the theme "It happened/I wanted it." The findings reveal that any simple determination of "agency" is negated by an appreciation of at least two elements: (1) their beliefs about life based in experience and (2) their perceptions about what there was to choose from. These elements raised questions about what it means to be agentic in a context of limited and constrained opportunities.

Briefly, the participants reported their belief that they should try to take control of events; indeed, experience had shown them that they are responsible for getting what they need. However, the participants also stated awareness of their limited ability to control events and to "pursue" certain goals. For example, Edouine expressed her desire to be a lawyer and said, "If it happens, it happens." While noting that she had been told to believe in herself or else it could not happen, she did not have any realistic plan to achieve this. In spite of this, she said she would try to remain optimistic.

These young women's discussions contained their reflections on the experiences that had taught them about what they could—and could not—expect in terms of support or opportunity. Four of the six participants talked about issues related to race, in particular, their experiences of racial discrimination. Although they said they tried to be optimistic about the future, they expressed doubt about the concrete prospects for educational and job success. Thus, their sense of agency is intimately connected to their sense of identity as young black women with unequal access to power and goods.

Any model of development that attempts to describe the lives of those outside the mainstream must acknowledge powerful structural and economic realities that constrain the possibilities for individual achievement. Such an approach must also deal with issues of power that may not always be apparent. In this case, what may look like passivity, or not having complete control, may also be a way to assert control. An expanded definition of agency must acknowledge how "one's ability to experience wants and goals and to take action to pursue them" is negotiated within constraining circumstances.

A Challenge to Traditional Distinctions Between Family and Work

The participants indicated that they planned to continue with their plans for school and work. Some said pregnancy offered a reason to recommit to education and had made their paths that much clearer. Although these statements may reflect a certain naïveté or optimism about the demands of parenting, their hopeful and pragmatic plans for school are supported by recent figures suggesting a large increase in the number of pregnant adolescents who continue their education. In discussing their plans for the future, the participants did not see childbearing as circumventing their plans for employment.

This may reflect patterns of family and childbearing that differ among members of different race and socioeconomic status groups. For example, Mirza's (1992) study of working-class girls in Britain found that black girls planned to combine childbearing and employment. This was in contrast to white working-class girls, who saw these as exclusive options and who planned to work outside the home only until they had children. Similarly, Collins's (1990) treatment of black motherhood notes that traditionally motherhood has not excluded working outside the home. Thus, there is a need to expand a conception of how motherhood, family, and work are combined.

As a related note, Hackett (1997) argues the importance of pursuing the relationships between women's identity development and career decisionmaking. She asserts the need to blur the marked distinction between career and identity development in order to reflect the inextricable link between personal and career lives and the need to incorporate new constructs in the study of women's career development, especially in research about women of color.

The Influence of Culture on the "Self" and Subjective Experience

The participants' discussions about life and their pregnancies indicated the potential influence of culture on their subjective experience. In particular, how they make sense of their pregnancies and identity within their cultural contexts may have an impact on their subjectivity. For example, the participants seemed acutely aware of others' and often their own previous judgments about teenagers, especially black teens, having babies. They seemed to struggle to incorporate the fact that they are pregnant in light of these beliefs; as Alicia said, "I used to look down on girls who used to get pregnant, especially the black females. That's what everybody expects from them, to have babies. . . . People think young black teenage girls are just out to get pregnant."

These comments support the idea that the social construction of black adolescent girls influences their development[4] and also suggests that they are not members of a single culture. They participate in at least two cultures (the dominant culture and the minority culture) and may struggle to negotiate between conflicting norms. Works by cultural psychologists, including Markus, Mullally, and Kitayama (1997), suggest the influence of culture on subjective experience and definitions of "self." Markus et al. (1997) suggest ways in which participation in sociocultural groups and contexts influences behavior and constitutes the self. They assert that "cultural contexts diverge not only in understandings of what the 'good' or moral self is thought to be, but in what type of entity or phenomenon the self is assumed to be" (p. 16).

The potential influence of African culture on black Americans' experience remains unclear; however, other cultural influences can be identified with more certainty. It seems the primary influence is that black girls grow up in an American culture that determines their experience. Growing up poor, and in a culture in which all women face gender inequality, also determines their experience. As Hill's (1999) work suggests, the influences of race, class, and gender are essential to the developmental experience of black American children. How these influences are incorporated into black American adolescent girls' sense of self and into subjective experience needs to be explored. The integration of these tasks and processes into a developmental model remains a challenge for the future.

Notes

1. See Damon (1996).
2. See Jessor, Colby, and Shweder (1996).
3. See also Flax (1993); Henriques, Hollway, Urwin, Venn, and Walkerdine (1994/1998); and Holland, Lachicotte, Skinner, and Cain (1998).
4. See Leadbeater and Way (1996).

References

Adams, G., Pittman, K., & O'Brien, R. (1993). Adolescent and young fathers: Problems and solutions. In A. Lawson & D. L. Rhode (Eds.), *The politics of pregnancy: Adolescent sexuality and public policy* (pp. 216–237). New Haven: Yale University.

Adler, N. E., & Tschann, J. M. (1993). Conscious and preconscious motivation for pregnancy among female adolescents. In A. Lawson & D. L. Rhode (Eds.), *The politics of pregnancy: Adolescent sexuality and public policy* (pp. 144–158). New Haven: Yale University.

Almeida, R. V., Woods, R., & Messineo, T. (1998). Child development: Intersectionality of race, gender, class and culture. *Journal of Feminist Family Therapy*, 10(1), 23–47.

Anderson, E. (1990). *Streetwise: Race, class and change in an urban community*. Chicago: University of Chicago Press.

______. (1993). Sex codes and family life among poor inner-city youths. In W. J. Wilson (Ed.), *The ghetto underclass: Social science perspectives* (pp. 76–95). Newbury Park, CA: Sage.

Arnett, J. J. (2000). Emerging adulthood: A theory of development from the late teens through the twenties. *American Psychologist*, 55(5), 469–480.

Banks, W. C., Ward, W. E., McQuater, G. V., & DeBritto, A. M. (1991). Are blacks external: On the status of locus of control in black populations. In R. L. Jones (Ed.), *Black psychology* (pp. 181–192). Berkeley, CA: Cobb & Henry.

Bell-Scott, P., & Guy-Sheftall, B. (1991). Introduction. In P. Bell-Scott, B. Guy-Sheftall, J. J. Royster, J. Sims-Wood, M. DeCosta-Willis, & L. P. Fultz (Eds.), *Double stitch: Black women write about mothers and daughters* (pp. 1–3). New York: HarperCollins.

Bell-Scott, P., & Taylor, R. L. (1989). Introduction: The multiple ecologies of black adolescent development. *Journal of Adolescent Research*, 4(2), 119–124.

Brewer, R. M. (1995). Gender, poverty, culture and economy: Theorizing female-led families. In B. J. Dickerson (Ed.), *African-American single mothers: Understanding their lives and families* (pp. 80–93). Thousand Oaks, CA: Sage.

Burden, D. S., & L. V. Klerman. (1984). Teenage parenthood: Factors that lessen economic dependence. *Social Work*, 29, 11–16.

Burton, L. M. (1990). Teenage childbearing as an alternative life course strategy in multigeneration black families. *Human Nature*, 1(2), 123–143.

Burton, L. M., Allison, K. W., & Obeidallah, D. A. (1995). Social context and adolescence: Perspectives on development among inner-city African-American teens. In L. J. Crockett & A. C. Crouter (Eds.), *Pathways through adolescence: Indi-*

vidual development in relation to social contexts (pp. 119–138). Mahwah, NJ: Erlbaum.

Burton, L. M., Obeidallah, D. A., & Allison, K. (1996). Ethnographic insights on social context and adolescent development among inner-city African-American teens. In R. Jessor, A. Colby, & R. A. Shweder (Eds.), *Ethnography and Human development*. Chicago: University of Chicago.

Carothers, S. C. (1990). Catching sense: Learning from our mothers to be black and female. In F. Ginsburg & A. L. Tsing (Eds.), *Uncertain terms: Negotiating gender in American culture* (pp. 232–247). Boston: Beacon Press.

Cauce, A. M., Hiraga, Y., Graves, D., Gonzales, N., Ryan-Finn, K., & Grove, K. (1996). African-American mothers and their adolescent daughters: Closeness, conflict and control. In B. J. Leadbeater & N. Way (Eds.), *Urban girls: Resisting stereotypes, creating identities* (pp. 100–116). New York: New York University Press.

Chodorow, N. (1978). *The reproduction of mothering*. Berkeley: University of California Press.

Coley, R. L., & Chase-Lansdale, P. L. (1998). Adolescent pregnancy and parenthood: Recent evidence and future directions. *American Psychologist*, 152–166.

Collins, P. H. (1990). *Black feminist thought: Knowledge, consciousness and the politics of empowerment*. Boston: Unwin Hyman.

______. (1991). The meaning of motherhood in black culture and black mother-daughter relationships. In P. Bell-Scott, B. Guy-Sheftall, J. J. Royster, J. Sims-Wood, M. DeCosta-Willis, & L. P. Fultz (Eds.), *Double stitch: Black women write about mothers and daughters* (pp. 42–60). New York: HarperCollins.

______. (1993). Shifting the center: Race, class, and feminist theorizing about motherhood. In G. Chang, L. R. Forcey, & E. N. Glenn (Eds.), *Mothering: Ideology, experience and agency* (pp. 45–65). New York: Routledge.

Crockett, L., & Crouter, A. C. (1995). *Pathways through adolescence: Individual development in relation to social context*. Hillsdale, NJ: Erlbaum.

Cross, W. E., Jr. (1991). *Shades of Black: Diversity in African-American Identity*. Philadelphia: Temple University Press.

Cross, W. E., Jr., Parham, T. A., & Helms, J. E. (1991). The stages of Black identity development: Nigrescence models. In R. L. Jones (Ed.), *Black psychology* (pp. 319–338). Berkeley, CA: Cobb & Henry.

Damon, W. (1996). Nature, second nature, and individual development: An ethnographic opportunity. In R. Jessor, A. Colby, & R. A. Shweder (Eds.), *Ethnography and human development* (pp. 460–474). Chicago: University of Chicago Press.

Dash, L. (1989). *When children want children: The urban crisis of teenage childbearing*. New York: William Morrow.

Davis, K., & Fisher, S. (1993). *Negotiating at the margins: Gendered discourses of power and resistances*. New Brunswick, NJ: Rutgers University Press.

Dickerson, B. J. (1995). *African-American single mothers: Understanding their lives and families*. Thousand Oaks, CA: Sage.

Dodson, L. (1998). *Don't call us out of name: The untold lives of women and girls in poor America*. Boston: Beacon Press.

Du Bois, W. E. B. (1989). *The souls of black folk.* New York: Penguin. (Original work published in 1903).

Earls, F. E., & Siegel, B. (1980). Precocious fathers. *American Journal of Orthopsychiatry*, 50, 469–480.

Elise, S. (1995). Teenaged mothers: A sense of self. In B. J. Dickerson (Ed.), *African American single mothers: Understanding their lives and families* (pp. 53–79).Thousand Oaks, CA: Sage.

Ely, M. (1984). Beating the odds: An ethnographic interview study of young adults from the culture of poverty. Paper presented at Seventh Annual Conference on English Education, New York University, NY.

Ely, M., Anzul, M., Friedman, T., Gardner, D., & Steinmetz, A. M. (1991). *Doing qualitative research: Circles within circles.* Bristol, PA: Falmer Press.

Erikson, E. (1968). *Identity: Youth and crisis.* New York: W. W. Norton.

Feldman, S. S., & Elliott, G. R. (1990). *At the threshold: The developing adolescent.* Cambridge: Harvard University Press.

Fine, M. (1989). Coping with rape: Critical perspectives on consciousness. In R. K. Unger (Ed.), *Representations: Social constructions of gender* (pp. 186–200). Amityville, NY: Baywood.

Fine, M., & Zane, N. (1991). Bein' wrapped too tight: When low income women drop out of high school. *Women Studies Quarterly*, 19(1, 2), 77–99.

Flax, J. (1993). *Disputed subjects: Essays on psychoanalysis, politics and philosophy.* New York: Routledge.

Fordham, S. (1993). "Those loud black girls": (Black) women, silence, and gender "passing" in the academy. *Anthropology and Education Quarterly*, 24(1), 3–32.

Franklin, D. L. (1987). Black adolescent pregnancy: A literature review. *Child and Youth Services*, 9, 15–39.

______. (1992). Early childbearing patterns among African-Americans: A sociohistorical perspective. In M. K. Rosenheim & M. F. Testa (Eds.), *Early parenthood and coming of age in the 1990s* (pp. 55–70). New Brunswick, NJ: Rutgers University Press.

Furstenberg, F. F., Brooks-Gunn, J., & Morgan, S. P.(1987). *Adolescent mothers in later life.* New York: Cambridge University.

Geronimus, A. T., & Korenman, S. (1990). *The socioeconomic consequences of teen childbearing reconsidered.* (Research Report No. 90-190). Ann Arbor: University of Michigan, Population Studies Center.

Gibbs, J. T. (1992). The social context of teenage pregnancy and parenting in the black community: Implications for public policy. In M. K. Rosenheim & M. F. Testa (Eds.), *Early parenthood and coming of age in the 1990s* (pp. 71–88). New Brunswick, NJ: Rutgers University Press.

Gilligan, C. (1982). *In a different voice: Psychological theory and women's development.* Cambridge: Harvard University Press.

Greene, B. (1990). Sturdy bridges: The role of African-American mothers in the socialization of African-American children. *Women and Therapy*, 205–225.

Guba, E. G., & Lincoln, Y. S. (1989). *Fourth generation evaluation.* Newbury Park, CA: Sage.

Gwaltney, J. L. (1980). *Drylongso: A self-portrait of Black America.* New York: Random House.

Hackett, G. (1997). Promise and problem in theory and research on women's career development. *Journal of Counseling Psychology*, 44, 184–188.

Hall, W. S., Freedle, R., & Cross, W. E., Jr. (1972). *Stages in the development of a black identity*. ACT Research Report 50. Iowa City: Research and Development Division, American Testing Program.

Harding, S. G. (1986). *The science question in feminism*. Ithaca: Cornell University Press.

______. (1991). *Whose knowledge? Whose science? Thinking from women's lives*. Ithaca: Cornell University Press.

Helms, J. E. (1990). *Black and white racial identity: Theory, research and practice*. New York: Greenwood.

Henriques, J., Hollway, W., Urwin, C., Venn, C., & Walkerdine, V. (1994/1998). *Changing the subject*. New York: Routledge.

Herman, J. L., & Lewis, H. B. (1984). Anger in the mother-daughter relationship. In T. Bernay & D. W. Cantor (Eds.), *The psychology of today's woman: New psychoanalytic visions* (pp. 139–163). Cambridge: Harvard University Press.

Hill, S. A. (1999). *African American children: Socialization and development in families*. Thousand Oaks, CA: Sage.

Hogan, D. P., & Kitagawa, E. M. (1985). The impact of social status, family structure, and neighborhood on the fertility of Black adolescents. *American Journal of Sociology*, 90, 825–855.

Holland, D., Lachicotte, W., Skinner, D., & Cain, C. (1998). *Identity and agency in cultural worlds*. Cambridge: Harvard University Press.

hooks, b. (1981). *Ain't I a woman? Black women and feminism*. Boston: South End Press.

Jacobs, J. L. (1994). Gender, race, class, and the trend toward early motherhood: A feminist analysis of teen mothers in contemporary society. *Journal of Contemporary Ethnography*, 22, 442–462.

Jessor, R. (1993). Successful adolescent development among youth in high-risk settings. *American Psychologist*, 48(2),117–126.

Jessor, R., Colby, A., & Shweder, R. A. (Eds.). (1996). *Ethnography and human development: Context and meaning in social inquiry*. Chicago: University of Chicago Press.

Jewell, K. S. (1992). Use of welfare programs and the disintegration of the black nuclear family. In R. Staples (Ed.), *The black family: Essays and studies* (pp. 319–326). Belmont, CA: Wadsworth.

Jordan, J. (1992) *Technical difficulties: African-American notes on the state of the union* (pp. 65–80). New York: Pantheon.

Kaplan, E. B. (1997). *Not our kind of girl: Unraveling the myths of black teenage motherhood*. Berkeley: University of California Press.

Ladner, J. A. (1971). *Tomorrow's tomorrow: The black woman*. New York: Doubleday.

Ladner, J. A., & Gourdine, R. M. (1984). Intergenerational teenage motherhood: Some preliminary findings. *SAGE: A Scholarly Journal on Black Women*, 1(2), 22–24.

Leadbeater, B. J., & Way, N. (1996). *Urban girls: Resisting stereotypes, creating identities*. New York: New York University Press.

Leslie, A. R. (1995). Women's life-affirming morals and the cultural unity of African peoples. In B. J. Dickerson (Ed.), *African-American single mothers: Understanding their lives and families* (pp. 80–93). Thousand Oaks, CA: Sage.

Lewis, M. (1997). *Altering fate: Why the past does not predict the future.* New York: Guilford Press.

Lincoln, Y. S., & Guba, E. G. (1985). *Naturalistic inquiry.* Newbury Park, CA: Sage.

Luker, K. (1996). *Dubious conceptions: The politics of teenage pregnancy.* Cambridge: Harvard University Press.

Mahoney, M. A., & Yngvesson, B. (1992). The construction of subjectivity and the paradox of resistance: Reintegrating feminist anthropology and psychology. *Signs: Journal of Women in Culture and Society,* 18(1), 44–73.

Markus, H. R., Mullally, P. R., & Kitayama, S. (1997). Selfways: Diversity in modes of cultural participation. In U. Neisser & D. Jopling (Eds.), *The conceptual self in context* (pp. 13–61). Cambridge: Cambridge University Press.

McCombs, H. G. (1986). The application of an individual/collective model to the psychology of black women. *Women and Therapy,* 5, 67–80.

McHale, S. M. (1995). Lessons about adolescent development from the study of African-American Youth: Commentary. In L. J. Crockett & A. C. Crouter (Eds.), *Pathways through adolescence: Individual development in relation to social contexts* (pp. 139–150). Mahwah, NJ: Erlbaum.

Merrick, E. N. (1995). *Negotiating the currents: Childbearing experiences of six lower socioeconomic status black adolescents.* Dissertation Abstracts, UMI.

______. (1999). Like "chewing gravel": On the experience of conducting qualitative research using a feminist epistemology. *Psychology of Women Quarterly,* 23(1), 49–59.

Mirza, H. S. (1992). *Young, female and black.* New York: Routledge.

Modell, J. (1996). The uneasy engagement of human development and ethnography. In R. Jessor, A. Colby, & R. A. Shweder (Eds.), *Ethnography and human development* (pp. 460–474). Chicago: University of Chicago Press.

Modell, J., & Goodman, M. (1990). Historical perspectives. In S. S. Feldman & G. R. Elliott (Eds.), *At the threshold: The developing adolescent* (pp. 93–122). Cambridge: Harvard University Press.

Morrison, D. M. (1985). Adolescent contraceptive behavior: A review. *Psychological Bulletin,* 98, 538–568.

Musick, J. S. (1993). *Young, poor and pregnant: The psychology of teenage motherhood.* New Haven: Yale University.

Nathanson, C. A. (1991). *Dangerous passage: The social control of sexuality in women's adolescence.* Philadelphia: Temple University Press.

National Center for Health Statistics. (1999). *Births: Final Data for 1997,* Vol. 47, No. 18.

National Vital Statistics Reports. (1999). Vol. 47, No. 25 (p. 10).

Parham, T. A. (1989). Cycles of psychological nigrescence. *Counseling Psychologist,* 17, 87–226.

Phinney, J. S., & Rosenthal, D. A. (1992). Ethnic identity in adolescence: Process, context, and outcome. In G. R. Adams, T. P. Gullotta, & R. Montemayor (Eds.), *Adolescent identity formation* (pp. 145–172). Newbury Park, CA: Sage.

Phoenix, A. (1993). The social construction of teenage motherhood: A black and white issue? In A. Lawson & D. L. Rhode (Eds.), *The politics of pregnancy: Adolescent sexuality and public policy* (pp. 74–97). New Haven: Yale University.

Polakow, V. (1993). *Lives on the edge: Single mothers and their children in the other America.* Chicago: University of Chicago Press.

Rhoden, J. L., & Robinson, B. E. (1997). Teen dads: A generative fathering perspective versus the deficit myth. In A. J. Hawkins & D. C. Dollahite (Eds.), *Generative fathering* (pp. 105–117). Thousand Oaks, CA: Sage.

Richardson, M. S. (1994). Agency/empowerment in clinical practice. *Journal of Theoretical and Philosophical Psychology*, 14(1), 40–49.

Riger, S. (1992). Epistemological debates, feminist voices: Science, social values, and the study of women. *American Psychologist*, 47, 730–740.

Robinson, T., & Ward, J. V. (1991). A belief in self far greater than anyone's disbelief: Cultivating resistance among African-American female adolescents. In C. Gilligan, A. G. Rogers, & D. Tolman (Eds.), *Women, girls and psychotherapy* (pp. 87–103). Binghamton, NY: Harrington Park Press.

Ruddick, S. (1993). Procreative choice for adolescent women. In A. Lawson & D. L. Rhode (Eds.), *The politics of pregnancy* (pp. 126–143). New Haven: Yale University Press.

Scott, K. Y. (1991). *The habit of surviving: Black women's strategies for life.* New Brunswick, NJ: Rutgers University Press.

Scott-Jones, D., Roland, E. J., & White, A. B. (1989). Antecedents and outcomes of pregnancy. In R. L. Jones (Ed.), *Black adolescents* (pp. 341–371). Berkeley, CA: Cobb & Henry Press.

Smith, E. J. (1982). The black female adolescent: A review of the educational, career and psychological literature. *Psychology of Women Quarterly*, 6, 261–288.

Sparks, E. E. (1996). Overcoming stereotypes of mothers in the African American context. In K. F. Wyche & F. J. Crosby (Eds.), *Women's ethnicities: Journeys through psychology* (pp. 67–86). Boulder, CO: Westview Press.

______. (1998). Against all odds: Resistance and resilience in African American welfare mothers. In C. G. Coll, J. L. Surrey, & K. Weingarten (Eds.), *Mothering against the odds: Diverse voices of contemporary mothers* (pp. 215–237). New York: Guilford Press.

Spradley, J. P. (1979). *The ethnographic interview.* New York: Holt, Rinehart & Winston.

Sternberg, R. J. (1986). A triangular theory of love. *Psychological Bulletin*, 93, 119–135.

Stewart, A. J. (1994). Toward a feminist strategy for studying women's lives. In C. E. Franz & A. J. Stewart (Eds.), *Women creating lives: Identities, resilience and resistance* (pp. 11–35). Boulder, CO: Westview Press.

Sue, D. W., & Sue, D. (1990). *Counseling the culturally different: Theory and practice.* New York: Wiley.

Sullivan, M. L. (1989). *"Getting paid": Youth crime and work in the inner city.* Ithaca: Cornell University.

Taylor, J. (1994). Adolescent development: Whose perspective? In J. M. Irvine (Ed.), *Sexual cultures and the construction of adolescent identities* (pp. 29–50). Philadelphia: Temple University Press.

Walker, A. (1982). One child of one's own: A meaningful digression within the work(s)—An excerpt. In G. T. Hull, P. Bell Scott, & B. Smith (Eds.), *But some of us are brave: Black women's studies* (pp. 37–44). New York: Feminist Press at The City University of New York.

Walkerdine, V. (1993). Beyond developmentalism? *Theory and Psychology,* 3(4), 451–469.

Ward, J. V. (1990). Racial identity formation and transformation. In C. Gilligan, N. P. Lyons, & T. J. Hamner (Eds.), *Making connections: The relational worlds of adolescent girls at Emma Willard School* (pp. 215–232). Cambridge: Harvard University Press.

Way, N., & Stauber, H. (1996). Are "absent fathers" really absent? Urban adolescent girls speak out about their fathers. In B. J. Leadbeater & N. Way (Eds.), *Urban girls: Resisting stereotypes, creating identities* (pp. 132–148). New York: New York University.

Weingarten, K., Surrey, J. L., Coll, C. G., & Watkins, M. (1998). Introduction. In C. G. Coll, J. L. Surrey, & K. Weingarten (Eds.), *Mothering against the odds: Diverse voices of contemporary mothers* (pp. 1–14) New York: Guilford Press.

Welsing, F. C. (1991). *The Isis Papers: The keys to the colors.* Chicago: Third World Press.

White, J. L. (1984). *The psychology of blacks: An Afro-American perspective.* Englewood Cliffs, NJ: Prentice-Hall.

Williams, T. W., & Kornblum, W. (1985). *Growing up poor.* Lexington, MA: Lexington Books.

Wilson, P. M. (1986). Black culture and sexuality. *Journal of Social Work and Sexuality,* 4, 29–47.

Wilson, W. J. (1980). *The declining significance of race: Blacks and changing American institutions.* Chicago: University of Chicago Press.

Wilson, W. J. (1987). *The truly disadvantaged: The inner city, the underclass, and public policy.* Chicago: University of Chicago Press.

Winfield, L. (1995). The knowledge base on resilience in African-American adolescents. In L. J. Crockett & A. C. Crouter (Eds.), *Pathways through adolescence: Individual development in relation to social contexts* (pp. 87–118). Mahwah, NJ: Erlbaum.

Zaslow, M. J., & Takanishi, R. (1993). Priorities for research on adolescent development. *American Psychologist,* 48(2), 185–192.

Ziegler, D. (1995). Single parenting: A visual analysis. In B. J. Dickerson (Ed.), *African-American single mothers: Understanding their lives and families* (pp. 80–93) Thousand Oaks, CA: Sage.

Index